Rebound 1981

MEDICAL TREATMENT OF THE DYING: MORAL ISSUES

edited by
MICHAEL D. BAYLES
and
DALLAS M. HIGH

G.K. HALL & COMPANY
SCHENKMAN PUBLISHING COMPANY

Copyright © 1978
Schenkman Publishing Company, Inc.
Cambridge, Massachusetts 02138

Library of Congress Cataloging in Publication Data

Bayles, Michael and High, Dallas M.
  Conference on Moral Issues of Medical Treatment of the
  Dying, University of Kentucky.
  Medical Treatment of the Dying: Moral Issues

  Bibliography
  1. Terminal care — Congresses. 2. Euthanasia — Congresses
  3. Physician and patient — Congresses
  I. Bayles, Michael D.   II. Title
  R726.8.C66 1974   174'.24.   76-41177
  ISBN 0-8161-2128-1

Printed in the United States of America

MEDICAL TREATMENT
OF THE
DYING:
MORAL ISSUES

Contents

Preface

The contributors to this volume represent different disciplinary backgrounds, and they are sensitive to the problems and views of those in other disciplines. Moreover, the diverse nature of the original audience* required that the papers be written in a clear, simple style without presupposing a technical background in any field. Consequently, the papers should be readable and intelligible to those without a philosophical or medical background. At the same time, they present most of the fundamental moral issues about medical care of the dying.

Due to the character of the essays included, we believe that this volume is suitable for a wide variety of uses. Anyone interested in the social problems of medical treatment for the dying may find it worth reading. It is intended for use in a variety of courses besides those specifically devoted to death and dying. For instance, it might be used in ethics courses to focus on concrete problems, or in social philosophy courses to illustrate the impact of technology on a significant aspect of society. Similarly, it might be used in courses in medical schools focusing on professional responsibility and the ethical issues of medical practice. We hope this volume serves to stimulate open and thoughtful interdisciplinary discussion of the issues involved.

*The papers, except those by the editors, were originally presented to a Conference on Moral Issues of Medical Treatment of the Dying held at the University of Kentucky and sponsored by its Graduate and Medical Schools. Approximately forty faculty from various disciplines met in October 1974 to discuss the issues. Because of the fruitful interchange they produced and the enduring nature of the issues, it is hoped that these papers will be considered a useful contribution to the field.

Introduction

The various professions — legal, educational, and medical — have always jealously guarded themselves from external evaluation and control. Standards of conduct and criteria for certification have been set by the professions themselves. Lawyers, teachers, and physicians have always considered themselves responsible for, but not accountable to, those they serve. In recent years, especially in the United States, there has been a marked trend towards making professionals more accountable to those they serve, which may be a part of a broader movement to protect consumers. This general trend has united with various recent developments in medicine to stimulate special attention to medical care of the dying.

The current widespread concern and interest in the medical profession and medical care must be viewed in historical perspective. Only during the last century or so have physicians had the knowledge and means to do much for their patients other than relieve symptoms and physical discomfort, and even that ability has advanced greatly. It was only during the latter part of the nineteenth century that the germ theory of disease was developed and antiseptics and anesthesia came into general use. Antibiotics are a twentieth century development. Hence, only in the last fifty years have physicians been able to offer patients a reasonable chance for effective treatment of the causes of diseases.

One effect of this scientific development has been to move death out of the home. Previously, most people died at home in the care of their family. Today, relatively few people die at home; instead, they die in hospitals. Due to the consciousness of the causes of death, the seriously ill are taken to hospitals which offer better facilities for treatment than the home. Hence, death has become physically removed from the context of everyday life, thereby assisting a common psychological tendency to avoid thought of death.

Even more recent scientific-technological advances have enabled physicians to preserve biological processes in circumstances previously undreamed of. A few years ago it was not possible to sustain cardiac and respiratory functions once they ceased. Now that process is possible with the use of "artificial" life support systems. For good reasons, physicians have historically been committed to struggle against death with all the resources at their command. This historical commitment has carried over into the modern context, so many physicians still use all the means at their disposal to continue life processes. The result is a curious anomaly from the standpoint of the patient: It is difficult to find a physician to provide treatment when one wants it, but even more difficult to get one to stop treatment of causes and instead focus on relief of symptoms and discomfort.

In addition, scientific-technological development has had an impact upon the patient-physician relationship. Fifty years ago the family physician was still the primary source of medical care. He treated all the ailments of all the members of the family, even doing most of the surgery. The family physician developed a general knowledge of the patient and his life circumstances. Today, because the increase in medical knowledge requires specialization, family physicians are rather uncommon. Medical service for a family is fragmented among various physicians — a pediatrician, a gynecologist, an internist, etc. In the hospital, medical teams are involved rather than one physician. Consequently, the close interpersonal relation between family physician and patient has largely disappeared since one physician is rarely responsible for the total patient care both in and out of the hospital.

Underlying the patient-physician relationship is a quasi-contractual legal-economic basis. The fee-for-services payment method essentially sets up contractual relationships between the patient and each of his physicians. The contractual nature of the relationship and the tort law of battery bring into prominence the consent of the patient. Under the fee-for-service system, the patient contracts for specific services and may supposedly limit the extent of services for which he contracts.

Moreover, a physician, especially a surgeon, may be liable for battery unless the patient has given his informed consent to all procedures performed.

However, as everyone knows from personal experience, one does not bargain with a physician over rates and specific services. The bargaining situation is weighted in favor of the physician. He has knowledge and expertise upon which the patient must rely. Moreover, the physician has a much larger group of potential patients than the would-be patient has range of potential physicians. In other unequal bargaining situations, e.g. travelers on common carriers, society has entered to regulate the contractual situation. Much of the current emphasis upon patient rights may perhaps be seen as an extension of such social control or regulation to the patient-physician relationship.

These changes in patient-physician relationships create enough difficulties for the ordinary person, but for a terminally ill patient they may be overwhelming. One must imagine a terminally ill patient in an intensive care unit of a hospital, without any family, facing a team of unknown doctors anxious to begin or continue various life-supporting treatments, bargaining over the precise limits of consent to treatment (and perhaps even charges). Consequently, in recent years, all these changes in the medical profession and patient-physician relationship have come to focus on the topic of medical treatment of the dying. The result has been widespread discussion and debate, and like any public discussion, has frequently been characterized by onesidedness, emotional appeal, and a lack of in-depth analysis of the issues and arguments. But also like other broad social issues, the problems are complex and the proper policies unclear.

The patient-physician relationship is one of four major themes or sets of issues found throughout the essays in this volume. It is the main topic of Tristram Engelhardt's paper. He contends that the fabric of rights and duties binding patients and physicians must be understood in their social setting. In particular, he contends that public financial support of medical research and training has changed modern medicine into a public enterprise. Consequently, patients may assert rights which are not based upon the contractual relationship but upon their status as members of society having civil rights.

The patient-physician theme is approached differently by James Toole, Robert Hudson, Dallas High, and Samuel Gorovitz. Toole discusses the responsibility thrown on a physician who must apply brain function indicators to determine whether a patient is dead. He also portrays several different approaches physicians take towards prolonging the life of their patients. Hudson argues that if euthanasia is to be practiced, physicians should not perform it because it might destroy patients' trust in them. Moreover, he recommends the development of a specially trained group of personnel to assist or replace physicians in dealing with the adjustment problems of dying patients. Yet, High argues that physicians should develop more skill and better regimens treating the debilitating and humiliating symptoms and effects of terminal illnesses. Finally, Gorovitz classifies the types of judgments physicians make in dealing with their patients and recommends that they should pay more attention to the well-being of the dying patient's family.

A second major theme addressed by many of these essays is the question of concepts and criteria of death and dying. Traditionally, cessation of respiratory and cardiac functions have been the indicators employed in death declaration. Technological developments have created difficulties: respiratory and cardiac functions may be continued when previously they would have ceased. Moreover, techniques have been developed to measure with varying reliability the cessation of brain activity. The practical significance of these developments came to the fore with the development of transplantation techniques. The shorter the time since respiratory and cardiac functions have ceased, the better suited are organs for transplantation. Hence, some people have argued that a person ought to be declared dead when it has been determined that the brain has ceased to function (so-called brain death) even though cardiac and respiratory functions continue. A number of states have adopted death statutes oriented to absence of brain function.

The essays by Gorovitz, Toole, High and Robert Veatch bear on this theme. Gorovitz offers a definition and criteria for properly regarding a person to be dying. He also argues that the concept of death is not value neutral; alternative definitions involve different evaluations of life. This point is aptly illustrated by Toole's presentation of a series of cases of brain damaged patients who might, depending upon the indicators used, be classified as dead. Indeed, he implicitly suggests that changing the indicators of death may be used as an alternative to euthanasia — instead of killing people they are merely classified as dead. High suggests that the concepts of life and death must be considered together and that the modern trend has been to quantify both and ignore the aspect of quality. He argues that both death declarations and care of dying persons are value-laden decisions about comprehensive entities. Finally, Robert Veatch considers the concept of natural death. He clarifies what may be meant by 'natural' and contrasts the concept of natural death with another conception in which no death is natural but all deaths are someone's fault.

A third major theme in the essays is the very popular quality of life issue, which the government is attempting to evaluate by developing a set of social indicators. However, 'quality of life' has several distinct senses depending upon the context in which it is used. In the environmental context, it pertains to the physical and cultural conditions in which one lives. In the medical context, it pertains to the capacities and experiences of the individual. The central issues concern (1) the standards for determining the quality of life and the quality needed to render life worth living, and (2) what medical treatments should be adopted with respect to a patient's quality of life.

The papers by Toole, Hudson, High, Michael Bayles and Veatch relate to this theme. Toole's discussion of the different types of brain damage which might justify classifying a person as dead may be viewed as concerned with the quality of life necessary to classify a person as alive. Hudson emphasizes the imprecision in various concepts related to the quality of life. In particular, he considers the concept of personhood and the attempts of "living wills" to specify the conditions in which life is no longer worth living. The treatment and care given a dying patient to sustain a high quality of life rather than merely prolong it is the major concern of High's paper. Michael Bayles sketches two standards which may be used in determining the quality of life and considers the different implications these standards have as to whether life is worth continuing. Finally, Veatch addresses the issue of quality of life in relation to efforts to extend the length of "natural life" and combat death. He criticizes various arguments which would oppose extending "natural life."

The fourth major theme concerns euthanasia and the termination of life-prolonging treatment. The issues involved have frequently been obscured by the use of persuasive definitions to support one side or another. Thus, while opponents of euthanasia may call it murder, proponents may extend 'euthanasia' to mean withholding or withdrawing treatment and direct killing, or speak euphemistically of assisted suicide. One task of philosophers is to cut through persuasive definitions to expose the underlying issues.

The topic is difficult and complex since there already exists in practice and in the common literature a number of distinctions. (1) One may distinguish conduct toward oneself from conduct toward others. If a person kills himself, it is usually called suicide; if the conduct resulting in death is that of another person, it is not. (2) Acts (performances, commissions) and forbearances (non-performances, omissions) may be distinguished. Shooting a person is an act; failing to provide any treatment is a forbearance. (3) One can generally distinguish between withholding (not starting) a treatment and withdrawing (stopping) it. (4) Some people distinguish ordinary and extraordinary or heroic treatments by determining whether they are customary and usual or by using other criteria. (5) One may distinguish between those acts of others done with, and those done without, the patient's consent. The appropriateness of these distinctions, of course, needs assessment.

Always moral issues should be distinguished from legal ones. For example, whether euthanasia (acts of killing by others for the sake of the "victim") should be legalized is a distinct issue from whether it is moral. Law and morality are not identical; there are different but overlapping reasons for their rules. The main legal issue concerns whether euthanasia should be legally permitted in regulated conditions. The moral issues are more numerous. One issue is whether there is any moral significance to be attached to the difference between acts and forbearances, i.e., a moral difference between killing and allowing to die. A second is whether the consent of the patient is morally necessary. A third is whether it is permissible to terminate extraordinary but not ordinary life-prolonging treatment.

Almost all the papers bear on this theme. Hudson considers the various difficulties in legalizing euthanasia upon request by the patient. John Ladd's entire essay is devoted to whether or not there is a moral difference between killing a patient and letting one die by ceasing life-prolonging treatment. He argues that the burden of proof is upon those who claim that acts are morally right or wrong rather than neutral. He then considers when a person is culpable for letting something happen and presents criteria for those forbearances which count as actions. Finally, he contends that both 'letting die' and 'killing' may apply to the same conduct and that killing is not unconditionally wrong.

The essay by Bayles adopts Ladd's contention that the burden of proof is upon those who would morally distinguish killing and allowing to die. After arguing against various attempts to defend a moral difference, he contends that in the absence of a moral difference the current practice of terminating treatment but not committing euthanasia of adults or infants is unjustified. He then argues that on any of three criteria as to when life is worth living, euthanasia is sometimes morally justified. However, Toole, Hudson, and High all suggest that euthanasia is rarely, if ever, appropriate. Gorovitz agrees with Ladd and Bayles that there is no moral difference between killing and permitting a patient to die by ceasing life-prolonging treatment, while Engelhardt argues that a dying patient's duties to others rarely provides a reason for constraining him to continue to live. Finally, Veatch suggests that emphasis upon natural death may lead to denying patients life prolonging treatment when they request it.

Thus, while the same four themes of the patient-physician relationship, the concept of death, the quality of life, and euthanasia weave through these essays, the authors often approach them from different perspectives or in different contexts. There is no doubt that the moral and policy issues related to medical treatment of the dying are many, complex, and involve fundamental values. The essays in this volume do not consider all of them. However, the authors raise basic issues and frequently put them in a novel perspective, providing the reader a basis upon which to reflect and arrive at his own views.

H. TRISTRAM ENGELHARDT, JR.

Rights and Responsibilities of Patients and Physicians

Patients and physicians are involved in a social fabric which includes medicine as a corporate endeavor, as well as society in general as a political structure. In the course of this paper, I will briefly describe the complexity of this fabric of rights and responsibilities which binds patients and physicians in the enterprises of medicine. I will argue that the physician-patient relationship is not merely one of patients and physicians. Rather, in order to understand the claims of rights and responsibilities as well as interests by patients and physicians, account must be taken of medicine as a profession and society as a political structure. In particular, most talk of patients' rights to health care, to knowledge of their prognoses, to refusing treatment, including life-prolonging treatment, can be fully accounted for only as claims to civil or political rights. In point of fact, such rights can rarely be secured contractually because patients are often too disadvantaged by disease itself, and because physicians have reasonable grounds for wanting to pursue treatment on their own terms. I will pursue these considerations with a focus on the dying patient, though the issues raised concern medicine generally.

In doing this, I will first sketch circumstances which usually disadvantage patients and review historically some of the central leitmotifs of physician-patient claims and counterclaims. I will then briefly analyze the nature of this fabric of rights and duties which binds patients and physicians. The thrust is that claims such as those to a "right to health care," or to a "right to death with dignity," develop out of a civil or political interest in medicine, a recent development which has in part transmogrified medicine. To put it another way, I will argue that a theoret-

9

ical account of such claims is best accomplished by an appeal to social or civil rights and duties which transcend individual contractual claims.

I. The Fabric

(1) *Disease and Death: The Setting of Medicine*

Death is a universal reality, a central structure of the human condition. The fact of death invites men to enlist physicians in the postponement of death and in making death easier. But, physicians obviously cannot prevent death; at best, they can substitute one cause of death for another, one time of death for another, one manner of death for another. Hence, ultimately medicine cares, it does not cure. The medical profession makes the passage through life more successful or more pleasant, often overcoming certain difficulties (i.e., curing particular diseases). But in the end, medicine must fail to cure, though there is no similar restraint on the possibilities for care. While death is beyond cure, the dying are usually capable of being cared for. Physicians, though, may be committed to cure when the patient is interested only in care. Moreover, there are circumstances which disadvantage the patient in choosing what care and/or cure he wishes, particularly if he is dying.

The physician-patient relationship is likely to be assumed under circumstances that compromise the integrity of the patient. Disease, injury, and the approach of death can disable and overwhelm freedom. At the very moments when much must be decided by the ill or dying person, he is often least able to decide with full competence. Disease not only places the patient at a general disadvantage, creating a need for the service of another, it also makes the patient dependent upon the physician for continued health and perhaps survival. Though patients may claim openness and participation in decisions concerning their own therapy as far as possible, such claims are countered by inescapable themes of paternalism, insofar as disease often involves a natural need for regression and dependence on the part of the patient. Concepts of informed consent seem to guide, yet these, too, always involve weighing different goods. There often exists a need *not* to be overly informed. For example, an anxious patient who has just sustained a serious myocardial infarction may not need, at that time, to be informed *precisely* of his prognosis because information might itself adversely change the prognosis. In short, one often enters into the arms of medicine as one might enter passionately into the arms of a lover — with great haste and need, but little forethought. And it often makes little sense to look for informed or voluntary consent in either case, if one wishes to understand consent in a rigorous and pure fashion. Patient and physician are thrown together because of the exigencies of nature. Other relations (e.g., the lawyer-client relation) rarely have their focus so immediately upon one's very presence in the world.

Disease, which is the occasion of the social interactions of medicine, imposes peculiar restrictions and reveals unique needs for trust and keeping trust. Though we all maintain basic rights, still we find ourselves in the grip of natural forces, the control of which often presupposes the intrusion of medicine in circumstances when our freedom is blunted.

Moreover, medicine, as all technical endeavors, has become increasingly less open to well-informed decision-making on the part of the general public. One of the most pervading consequences of modern technological society is the social distribution of knowledge (i.e., groups of experts possess various portions of society's store of knowledge; the knowledge explosion precludes all from full possession of our current stock of knowledge) [1] which prevents fully informed individual, and to some extent societal, decisions and consent concerning the directions of medicine. The accrual of a special stock of skills and knowledge by a particular group of individuals, with consequent peculiar social duties, rights, powers, and expectations, in part defines medicine as a profession and distinguishes the physician from the layman, his actual or potential patient. It establishes not only divisions of labor but of power due to the possession of special knowledge bearing on the life and death of laymen. It also establishes a social sub-group defined by its interest in the preservation and maintenance of its skills and knowledge, and thus by special interests and goals.

However, to talk of rights and responsibilities of patients and physicians in the absence of any reference to the goals of society in general or of the medical profession in particular, is to prescind artificially from the actual context of patients and physicians. Physicians have civil duties *to* society and *to* their profession *regarding* patients that extend beyond the rights that patients have with respect to physicians.[2] Physicians have a duty to society to report communicable diseases, for example, which is not a duty to any particular patient. Moreover, patients possess certain duties *to* society *regarding* physicians and the medical professions which they do not have strictly to physicians. Patients with communicable diseases have a duty to society to follow the advice of their physicians with regard to preventing their spread.

Further, modern medicine is the creation of society; public investment in the education of physicians and medical research has produced it. Medicine has become part of society's explicit political response to the general predicament of man. That is, society has begun to invest in and use medicine for the general political purposes of the community. Private individuals no longer provide the major support for medical research and education.[3] Rather, medicine has become a social or civil instrument, and in this sense has become socialized. Medicine has been employed to affect the conditions of society, e.g., change infant mortality rates, enable a population explosion, provide contraception, make life in cities possible without frequent fatal epidemics, etc., and it has thereby become an instrument of society in the sense of a publicly supported means of effecting publicly chosen goals.

This thesis of the social or civil nature of medicine is stronger and more complex than the more general maxim of "he who pays the piper calls the tune." The relation of society and medicine is no longer merely a contractual one. The compass of modern medicine is a political creation. As a result, physicians accrue both rights and duties. They acquire duties to society regarding particular patients. Members of society also acquire social duties to have immunizations, blood tests, special examinations for certain occupations (food handlers, airplane pilots, etc.). These are civil duties of "patients" to society regarding medicine. It is in this broader social context that citizens have a civil right to health care. Their right is one from society regarding medicine, one in virtue of modern medicine existing as a social product. We will return to this issue when discussing the socialization of medicine.

(2) Historical Leitmotifs

In talking about physicians and patients, one must view the issues in terms which transcend relations between particular physicians and patients, and concern general social or civil structures. Further, the interests and enterprises shared by physicians and patients is such that duties and rights are never unilateral; rather, they are mutually implicatory and asymmetrical. Patients trade money and freedom for care and cure. A brief sketch of attitudes expressed in the Hippocratic corpus and the first A.M.A. code is illustrative.

The Hippocratic corpus is a diverse collection of writings on medicine, which has been imputed to Hippocrates (circa 460-379 B.C.), but which reflects more than one tradition. It contains at least four treatises with significant focus on values in medicine: "The Oath," "Law," "The Physician," and "Decorum." Though other treatises in the corpus refer to medical ethical issues, only these have a primary focus on the ethical conduct of medicine. They are central to the lore of medicine. The Oath in particular concerns both physician and patient rights.[4] From physicians, the Oath requires loyalty and support of their teachers and an esoteric attitude towards medical knowledge. Medical knowledge was to be communicated to the initiate but not to others, an attitude still prevalent today. Patient-directed concerns included the duty to give proper treatment, to avoid taking advantage of the special intimacies of the physician-patient relationship and, in particular, to maintain confidentiality.[5]

The Oath evidences a recognition of the peculiar nature of the physician-patient relationship as established on the basis of the vicissitudes of nature. Because of a person's vulnerability to disease, he is forced to the physician for aid. The physician, moreover, is a part of a community of physicians. Patients, on the other hand, apart from some social recognition, are not a social body but merely an aggregate of persons gathered together by chance, indeed, bad luck. By the nature of the circumstances and the relationship, the patient is disadvantaged, if not disabled, and is at the mercy of the physician. Beyond that, the process of cure requires disclosure of the patient's body, his way of life, and his habits to the physician. In the process, the physician gains a unique and privileged knowledge of the patient. But the intimacy is one-sided. The physician is not constrained to reciprocate except with competent therapy, confidentiality, and restraint from using the relationship for clearly self-interested motives. The Oath requires the physician to be circumspect and not to seduce his patients.

To put it another way, the Oath recognizes that the physician and the patient meet in circumstances structured by the difficulties of the patient and by the art of medicine. There are always at least four elements involved: the physician, the patient, the disease, and medicine. In modern communities, one must add a fifth element: society in the form of a political structure. As stated in the Hippocratic corpus, "The art has three factors, the disease, the patient, the physician. The physician is the servant of the art. The patient must co-operate with the physician in combating the disease." [6] The physician, as servant of the art (i.e., the profession of medicine), brings interests peculiar to himself: the goals and pleasures of medicine. An art well practiced is an end in itself, which is no less the case with medicine. Diagnosis and consequent explanation and prediction, or prognosis, are intellectual goals which can lead to social approval even in the absence of therapy. And again, importantly, the corpus suggests that the physician's duty regarding the patient is to the profession: "The physician is the servant of the art." [7]

This fabric of interests (i.e., those of patients, of individual physicians, and of the profession of medicine) structured the development of the present concept of medical ethics. In America, the historical development shows the evolution of a fabric of social concerns. Initial interest in medical ethics centered upon establishing the etiquette of proper medical practice.

This emphasis is reflected in the "Boston Medical Police" of 1808, and the numerous early codes of "Medical Etiquette" which followed.[8] These codes were in great proportion focused on regulating consultations, interactions of physicians, and setting a schedule of fees.

The current term "medical ethics" gained currency and one of its meanings was fixed in the United States when the American Medical Association adopted its "Code of Medical Ethics" at its first meeting in May, 1847.[9] This code dealt explicitly with duties of different kinds: duties of physicians to patients, of patients to physicians, of physicians to their profession and fellow physicians, of the profession to society, and of society to the profession. Duties of physicians to patients included offering treatment to the ill; keeping confidentiality; giving adequate care; not giving gloomy prognoses (in particular, not informing a patient of his impending death); not abandoning a patient when only care, not cure, was possible; and consulting other physicians when necessary. In other words, the physician was to give care and treatment while keeping trust with his patient and recognizing his own limitations. The patient, on the other hand, was to respond by selecting only bona fide physicians (not quacks), being open and complete in giving the history of his diseases, following the orders of the physician "promptly and implicit[ly]" and not leaving one physician for another without first giving the reasons for this action, etc. Patients, in short, were to submit almost unquestioningly to the treatment of their physicians. In addition, as in the Oath, there was a recognition of duties of physicians to their fellows and to the profession itself. Finally, there was an acknowledgment of duties of physicians to society and of society to physicians and medicine: physicians were seen to have an obligation to aid the development of social policy in matters of public health, while the community was seen to have the duty to encourage and facilitate medical education, etc.

In short, the history of Western medicine places the physician-patient relationship in the context of the community of physicians, if not that of society generally. Finally, even in the absence of historical argument, there is a somewhat obvious development of the social nature of medicine. In Greek times, the author of "Law" could assert: "Medicine is the only art which our states have made subject to no penalty save that of dishonour...."[10] But in 1847, the same year in which the A.M.A. code was written, Salomon Neumann was arguing for "the social nature of the healing art."[11] And shortly thereafter, that argument was assumed by Rudolf Virchow, who finally contended that medicine should deal with the basic laws of social structure.[12] Any account of patient and physician rights and responsibilities must therefore sort out different levels and kinds of claims and counterclaims, social and individual.

II. The Meaning of the Fabric

How then are we to understand the complex fabric of rights and duties binding patients and physicians? What is its nature? The conclusion seems to be that the rights and duties are not only complex but heterogeneous in nature. Some historically more basic ones are in part contractual and in part imposed by the circumstance that most patients are in some sense disabled. The rights and duties are contractual in the sense of arising out of the therapeutic contract between physicians and patients: the patient can always refuse any treatment, or the treatment of a particular physician, though the consequences may be severe. Physicians can, on the other hand, refuse to treat particular patients, but with less dire consequences. A physician is not usually in as pressing a need for a patient, at a particular time, as a patient is for a physician. Yet, there are circumstances when the patient determines the direction of the relationship rather than leaving it to a physician's judgment, as for example when a rhinoplasty or an abortion is sought. But the constraints of nature (e.g., fever, fear, delirium, pain, simple weakness), constraints of the social distribution of knowledge, and the interests of the profession of medicine in pursuing its own goals usually curtail full patient knowledge about the significance of treatment and thus curtail participation in determining the course of treatment. Physicians as members of an independent enterprise may simply refuse to make such participation an element of the therapeutic relationship.

Thus to a great extent the relation of physicians and patients arises out of the state of things, just as marriage arises out of the mutual needs of the sexes, or a family out of the mutual needs and abilities of its members. When ill, one is often simply dependent on a physician, as a small child is on its parents; the physician's paternalism is in this sense a natural one born out of the constraints of nature. That is, in this context, physician and patient rights arise as much out of the status of the individuals involved as out of any contract.

The contractual relations of physicians and patients are thus usually unequal because patients enter such contracts under duress, while physicians are supported by a strong profession with independent goals. How then are we to understand the character and place of patient rights such as those of the Patient's Bill of Rights of the American Hospital Association? What is the basis of claims such as "the right to obtain from [one's] physician complete current information concerning [one's] diagnosis, treatment, and prognosis in terms the patient can be reasonably expected to understand [or] when it is not medically advisable to give such information to the patient [to have that] information . . . made available to an appropriate person in [the patient's] behalf," or "the right to refuse treatment to the extent permitted by law . . ."?[13] These strong statements of patient rights imply a parity between physician and patient not usually possible in the situations under which therapeutic contracts, physician-patient relationships, are developed. Nor are such claims to rights claims to contractual rights, for it is difficult to argue that physicians would generally agree to physician-patient relationships that are contrary to the interests of physicians in care and cure. Further it is difficult to see how patients have a prima facie right such that physicians would have a duty to agree to therapeutic contracts which physicians find to collide with the aims and purposes of medicine.

(1) Patient Interests and Rights Versus the Physician

Patients have an interest in gaining cure and care, and in avoiding loss of freedom or privacy. But since disease and death

involve partial or total loss of liberty, patients are usually willing to cede some freedom in order to maintain liberty from
illness and death. Claims to privacy are often withdrawn in
order to secure cure and care. Conflicts arise when a patient
decides that the sacrifice of freedom and privacy is not justified
by the cure or care offered, while others, physicians in particular, hold such cure or care to be in that person's best interests.
Such conflicts are likely to arise in cases of incurable diseases
and are often articulated in terms of rights to refuse treatment,
especially extraordinary treatment. Conflicts also arise in terms
of claims that it is in the best interests of a patient not to know the
true severity of his illness.

The strongest general arguments on behalf of the patient are
those with regard to the patient as a free agent. If respect is due to
persons as free agents, then to preempt another's freedom to
choose in his own behalf is precisely not to treat that person as
free. Freedom to decide one's own best interests is, in the end,
the core of self-determination. Yet, there is a dilemma, for it is
illness and approaching death which are likely to overwhelm a
patient and make self-determination difficult, if not impossible.
The issue of patient rights is then, as has been argued, to be
weighed against a paternalism required because of the intru-
sions of disease. It has been accepted by some (though more so in
the past than in the present) that the patient's right to consent to
his treatment and to knowledge concerning its significance is
suspended when such knowledge and decisions might unduly
stress the patient. I have in mind a situation in which a physician
would say to a patient, "If you want me to treat you, trust me,
follow my orders, I will take care of you, there is nothing more
you need to know about your heart attack than that I will treat
you well and in your best interests."[14]

But not only does the patient have a right to expect that the
physician will act only in the patient's best interest, he also has a
right to attempt to negotiate with the physician the bounds of
such paternalism. Yet when such paternalism is accepted by the
profession of medicine and by society as usually being beneficial, it becomes a generally established social practice. In such
circumstances, what claims can the patient succeed in making

against medicine? Or, rather, how can such claims be framed? Medicine as an independent social enterprise sets its own standards, and the patient can at best demand that the physician not abuse the powers that come into his hands as a result of the physician's following the established mode of giving treatment. All things being equal, persons may become physicians in order to cure and care, and may hold that (1) this is their prime goal, and (2) too much information conveyed to the patient may thwart that goal. Insofar as medicine can act as an independent social enterprise, physicians may simply say — take it or leave it.

The situation is one in which the physician can see himself as the agent of cure and care, not the agent of the patient, who must therefore accept cure and care on the physician's terms. Physicians, moreover, can bolster such stances by appeals that anything less than resolute, unwavering dedication to cure will (1) cause patients to be abandoned prematurely as hopeless when more resolute physicians would have effected a cure, and (2) lead patients to lose confidence in their physicians. That is, physicians can appeal to a policy of "dedication to cure at all costs" as being the best policy for most patients in the long run.

There are two axes along which the success of such arguments can be plotted. One is the mental competence of the patient and the second is the likelihood of survival given persistent therapy. Thus, the more a patient is overwhelmed by the disease process itself and the greater the likelihood of cure given persistent therapy, the easier it is to justify a physician's paternalism by an argument in terms of those best interests which the patient himself would pursue, were he clear of intellect. One should imagine here a patient suffering miserably from a painful but easily curable disease who is ready to abandon all hope. Given the pain and exhaustion involved in illness, a patient is liable to despair prematurely.

This is similar to the account of Odysseus given by Dworkin. Odysseus' crew is justified in not freeing him from the mast, even if he so requests, because that was the reason he had himself bound in the first place — so he could resist the Sirens.[15] Often an argument similar to that of Odysseus' crew can be made by the physician — namely, to secure the patient against the

Sirens of depression and despair. In such cases, the physician's dedication to cure and care and against allowing euthanasia or suicide provides a "social insurance" policy.[16] There is a good case for the physician's treating as far as possible and being as persuasive as possible in attaining the patient's consent to treatment, *when* there is a reasonable chance for cure of a patient who is not in a position to decide on the significance of his chances. The physician can then presume that when the patient entered into the physician-patient relationship, he wanted the assurance of such action and gave implicit consent to "benign coercion."

Claims to such paternalism, though, are weakened when the patient is relatively clear of mind and his chances of survival are minimal, if not nil. In the imminence of death, neither the patient nor society can gain anything from further prolongation of life. In such cases, the patient may make a presumptively valid claim that any and all further treatment should cease and he be free to commit suicide. I will leave the issue of assisted suicide in the imminence of death, i.e., euthanasia, unexamined because it raises more issues than are pertinent here. It is enough here to indicate that the imminence of death, along with physical incapacitation, excuses one from most duties. In short, there rarely are good grounds under which a dying person with severe physical incapacitation can be constrained to live further because of duties to others or society.[17] It should be noted that this point is made without reference to extraordinary or ordinary means of therapy: when there is no need to constrain the present freedom of an individual as a rational insurance that in the future he can act freely, constraint is not justified. While one often prevents irrevocable decisions that would seriously undercut one's ability to choose freely in order to maintain freedom in the future, the imminence of death removes the need for such calculations.

So-called living wills, instructions to one's physician regarding what the physician's actions should be if the patient is incapacitated, are designed to provide a clear notion of the will of the patient in some of these circumstances. Living wills are doubly conditional physician-patient contracts. Most physician-patient relationships are conditional upon the continued consent of both partners. A living will (among other things) can explicitly condition the patient's consent upon a significant chance of survival as a conscious agent. So, for example, a living will could provide that, if in the future the patient is unconscious with no likely chance of regaining consciousness, there would be no consent to further treatment.

But there are other grounds in terms of which medicine and physicians may still find reasons to constrain patients to submit to treatment, even when there is little likelihood of cure and it only prolongs dying. Physicians might argue, for example, that such a course provides a patient comfort built on a hope, albeit a vain hope. Further, physicians might hold that one should never stop treatment as long as there is any hope, however remote. Such attitudes are of long standing in American medicine, especially with regard to the physician never being the person to tell a patient that his condition is fatal. "For the physician should be the minister of hope and comfort to the sick; that, by such cordials to the drooping spirit, he may smooth the bed of death, revive expiring life, and counteract the depressing influence of those maladies which often disturb the tranquillity of the most resigned in their last moments. The life of a sick person can be shortened not only by the acts, but also by the words or the manner of the physician. It is, therefore, a sacred duty to guard himself carefully in this respect, and to avoid all things which have a tendency to discourage the patient and to depress his spirits." [18]

The point is that the physician should attempt to act in the best interests of the patient, which include living as long and as free from suffering and anxiety as possible. This view of course conflicts with the notion that some patients may choose a life lived on their own terms, even if shorter and more marked by anxiety derived from a true knowledge of their impending death. The issue is the extent to which a patient, in particular a dying patient, has rights to full knowledge concerning his condition and to participate in decisions concerning his treatment.

On the other hand, the physician has independent claims and interests. The physician has presumably entered into the practice of a particular profession because he or she enjoys the activities of that art and science. He has an interest and indeed a *prima facie* right not to be forced to do things which he holds to be against good medical judgment, thereby making a claim for intellectual integrity. In fact, the physician can make such strong claims as, "If you want me to treat you, then you will have to follow my directions for therapy." The physician has a proper interest in the patient following the prescribed treatment beyond merely having the patient pay his bills. The physician makes a claim for the integrity of his art and science as a condition of his practice. Finally, one should remember that medicine can be practiced independently of goals of cure, as the history of therapeutic nihilism attests.[19] Medicine can be satisfying to the physician as a purely intellectual undertaking, the parody of which are statements such as "the operation was a success but the patient died." But even in such statements of derision, a legitimate claim is made to pursue an art with integrity of judgment and purpose.

Further, the profession of medicine presupposes the acquisition of skill and its transmission from one practitioner to another. Insofar as medicine has as its goal the cure of disease and the care of man in illness and dying, and insofar as medicine always fails to cure and care fully, there arises a basic nisus to research, observation, and the development of further knowledge of skills in treatment and care. Patients are thus also subjects of at least clinical observations. They are always possible contributors to medical knowledge as well as patients, recipients of medical care. Further, as a science and technology, medicine has its own independent interest in knowledge which can exceed that of society — to which past disapproval of anatomical dissection and present opposition to the study of *in vitro* fertilization attest.[20]

Unlike society at large, the medical profession has a special investment in the goals of medical progress. Increase in medical knowledge and technology represents an increase in the abilities and prestige of the medical profession and its individual members. It represents, as well, the achievement of an intrinsic goal of medicine: the better understanding and treatment of disease. Though for society in general, a certain high level of health might be sufficient, medicine always has an implicit commitment to advance and, therefore, to further experimentation and investment of resources in the expansion of medical knowledge and technology. There is a conflict implicit in this goal, for the progress of medical knowledge requires the use of large numbers of human beings in medical research and experimentation. In particular, these internal interests of medicine can lead to conflicts with medicine's more general interests in cure and care. These conflicts can become acute with regard to special groups such as the dying, who may be asked to submit to research which may not benefit their cure or care, though the dying may vainly and falsely so hope.

In summary, against these claims by physicians and the medical profession, patients can make only relatively weak counterclaims, if the physician-patient relationship is only a narrowly construed contractual one. While patients can refuse to contract with particular physicians, they may be forced by disease to contract with physicians on terms for the most part set by nature and by the paternalistic judgments of medicine. A patient can demand the care and cure and to withdraw at will from the relationship, but he cannot, without further negotiation, demand that treatment, if given, be given in any way except in terms of the medical judgment of the treating physician. That is, the physician as expert makes a claim to know best and, if engaged, to be allowed to act upon that better knowledge. There is also a paternalistic element to this position, that at a future time (i.e., after being cured), the patient will agree that it was good to have been induced to follow the physician's advice. Thus, modern claims such as those to a right to health care or to full knowledge concerning the course of one's treatment and therefore full participation in decisions concerning it, must arise, if they are to arise at all, from sources other than a physician-patient contract.

(2) The Socialization of Medicine

My use of the phrase, "socialization of medicine," is somewhat idiosyncratic; it is meant to focus on a general shift in the significance of patient rights with regard to medicine. In particular, the social nature of medicine augments the otherwise circumscribed rights of patients, providing a context in terms of which the physician-patient contract can be renegotiated, giving the patient more parity with the physician by sustaining his claims to knowledge and decision, even if sustaining such claims is not conducive to effective treatment.

The point is that, because of societal investment in the development of medical research and education, public health care programs, and individual health care (e.g., Medicare), medicine has become an element of social or civil policy. Medicine, once an enterprise of private citizens, has now become an extension of those citizens through the development of medicine within a political structure. The force of this development is that medicine as a social or political enterprise can legitimately be required to temper its interests in cure and care and make them accord with basic claims of citizens to self-determination and choice. In this sense, rights to health care and patient bills of rights are of civil rights, rights which accrue to an individual in virtue of his membership in a political structure of a certain character. One begins thus to speak of a new quality of patient freedom, even though its quantity, its scope, can never (because of the restraints of disease and the social distribution of knowledge) be comparable to that of the physician. Patient bills of rights involve bringing the pursuit of cure and care on medicine's terms into a social context of basic non-medical concerns for self-determination, so that such concerns are less likely to be overridden.

It is worth remarking again that the patient is probably most disadvantaged in the imminence of death, when there will not be a future time in which the social insurance of a medical paternalism could be evaluated by that patient. Moreover, choices of the point at which further treatment ceases to make sense are probably much more an issue of what makes sense for that patient; they are more idiosyncratic and less amenable to judgments made on the basis of medical paternalism. The point at which further pain incurred to prolong life is no longer justified by the quality of life achieved is an issue best determined by the person suffering the pain and living that life. One might think here of a patient with disseminated carcinoma, deciding against further treatment on the basis that further investment of pain and effort is not worth the likely return. Again, if present paternalistic constraint is to be justified on the basis of protection of future freedom of the patient, the justification fails in the case of the dying patient. There will be no future of any material significance. The issue here is in part that of allowing the patient to decide what counts as a meaningful extension of his future, given the fact of his imminent death. The patient here would need a clear notion of his prognosis to decide intelligently when further treatment is no longer justified. Such claims, though, can conflict with an interest physicians have in deciding when further treatment should be foregone. However, the social nature of modern medicine provides a political context in which such claims by patients can be raised as general civil rights and thus as prior yet complementary to any particular physician-patient contracts. Such claims by patients are basically claims to a general civil right to liberty — even to the point of caprice.

The socialization of medicine paradoxically implies both less and more freedom. On the one hand, it provides an arena in which general claims to greater parity in physician-patient relationships can be made. That is, patients as citizens can constrain medicine, an enterprise of their society, to allow patients to share in the responsibility for treatment and diagnosis. On the other hand, the socialization of medicine (i.e., the placing of medicine within a political structure and thus in terms of civil policies) implies that an element of general societal concern will extend to general treatment of the population — fluoridation and chlorination of water supplies, the requirement of vaccinations, etc. The socialization of medicine can not only give all persons a civil right to health care and to participation in decisions concerning their treatment, but it can also impose on them civil duties to participate in health maintenance, even in programs which cannot be directly in their self-interest (e.g., rubella vaccinations). In short, the socialization of medicine involves the placing of individual concerns about disease, health, care and cure in terms of general civil goals. It provides a domain within which talk about general rights and duties with regard to health care can take place.

In particular, talk of patients' rights to health care, to full knowledge concerning their prognosis, to terminating life-prolonging therapy, can gain a meaning in terms of duties to society by medicine regarding those patients. They can be viewed as rights from society, as a political institution, regarding medicine. It is not as if a particular physician had a duty to accept a particular patient as his and discharge his general duty to provide health care in the instance of that particular patient. Nor is it really the case that, all things being equal, a physician, qua physician, has a duty to let a patient determine the criteria for informing the patient concerning his prognosis or for terminating his treatment. It is rather, I suggest, that such issues arise in terms of the scope of the patients' basic civil rights. Otherwise puzzling talk about rights to health care can thus be given a sense, a social one. Patients' rights, including the rights of the dying patient, are, if they are to be rights at all, civil rights. They are claims that must be formally recognized by society.

This development should not be unexpected. The claim of patients to bills of rights is the claim to have the right to develop a social policy which will structure the practice of medicine. Claims to patient rights and liberties grow out of general civil claims to rights and liberties, which is to say that patients form the larger society within which physicians and medicine are finally placed. Until general society comes to terms with the rights of patients, patients suffer from an anomie, to which physicians as members of a uniting enterprise (i.e., medicine) are not subject. Patients are merely isolated patients until society addresses the status of medicine and patients. Only then can a patient receive special standing as a free citizen with rights with respect to health care.

This point is not unlike that made by Plato concerning the difference between free and slave physicians. "A physician of this kind [a slave] never gives a servant any account of his complaint, nor asks him for any . . . [But], the free practitioner . . . treats [his patients'] diseases by going into things thoroughly from the beginning in a scientific way, and takes the patient and his family into his confidence." [21] To develop this point with broad brushstrokes yet one further step, in a society of free men, claims can be made not only to a right to knowledge concerning one's illness and to a right to consent knowingly to therapy, but to a right to refuse life-prolonging therapy as well. Concepts of death with dignity thus become more the notion of a death chosen under circumstances most in accord with the wishes of the patient as a free citizen. Since disease and the imminence of death can make full, voluntary, and informed consent impossible, such participation becomes an ideal more than a completely realizable goal. Attempts to articulate patients' bills of rights and to provide for living wills are attempts to extend personal freedom into the relationships of physicians and patients, to provide ideals for citizen participation. Such bills of rights act to bring elements of general human freedom into circumstances otherwise structured only by the forces of nature and the interests of medicine. In particular, it may be necessary for society to protect a patient's right to choose death rather than a prolonged dying that an over-dedication to cure might entail. One sees at play here a general role of political structures, namely, to place the legitimate concerns of special interest groups within the context of the interests of society at large. Medicine is the special interest group of cure and care. However, citizens may not always have an interest in cure and may instead desire care on their own terms.

NOTES

I am indebted to Laurence McCullough for criticism and discussion of the ancestral drafts of this paper.

1. Alfred Schutz and Thomas Luckmann, *The Structures of the Life-World*, trans. Richard M. Zaner and H. Tristram Engelhardt, Jr. (Evanston: Northwestern University Press, 1973), pp. 324-326.

2. A good discussion of duties one has to A regarding B is given by Marcus G. Singer in his article "On Duties to Oneself," *Ethics* 69 (1959): 204.

3. Report by the Committee on the Financing of Medical Education of the Association of American Medical Colleges, "Current Funding Patterns: Medical School Programs," *Journal of Medical Education* 49 (1974): 1097-1102.

4. The document, though, is probably of Pythagorean origin, representing the views of that particular philosophico-religious sect and not that of the general medical community of the time. Ludwig Edelstein, *The Hippocratic Oath: Text, Translation and Interpretation*, Supplement No. 1, *The Bulletin of the History of Medicine* (Baltimore: The Johns Hopkins Press, 1943), pp. 14-38.

5. Further, in a somewhat religious tone, the Oath required one to conduct one's medical practice in purity and holiness. It was this latter leitmotif which led to its unique proscriptions of abortion, euthanasia, and surgery — practices which violated Pythagorean religious prohibitions, but which were otherwise fairly widely practiced in the Graeco-Roman world prior to the Christian era. I will pass over these latter issues, which are still primarily religious, and focus on the broader context of physician and patient interests.

6. Epidemics I, xi. *Hippocrates*, Vol. 1, trans. W. H. S. Jones (London: William Heinemann Ltd., 1923), p. 165.

7. *Ibid.*

8. Donald E. Konold, *A History of American Medical Ethics, 1847-1912* (Madison: The State Historical Society of Wisconsin for the Department of History, University of Wisconsin, 1962), p. 2.

9. *Ibid.*, p. 9, and *Code of Medical Ethics Adopted by the American Medical Association* (New York: New York Academy of Medicine, 1848).

10. Law i. *Hippocrates*, Vol. 2, p. 263.

11. Solomon Neumann, *Dieöffentliche Gesundheitspflege und das Eigenthum* (Berlin: Adolph Riess, 1847), p. 65.

12. Rudolf Virchow, "Uber die Standpunkte in der wissenschaftlichen Medicin," *Archiv für pathologische Anatomie und Physiologie* 70 (1847): 1-10.

13. American Hospital Association, "Statement on a Patient's Bill of Rights, Affirmed by the Board of Trustees, November 17, 1972," *Hospitals* 47 (February 16, 1973): 41.

14. One should remember that such bold paternalism is almost all medicine had to offer until the late nineteenth century. Further, such a demeanor, when accepted, probably itself has a beneficial, placebo effect.

15. Gerald Dworkin, "Paternalism," *Monist* 56 (1972): 77.

16. *Ibid.*, p. 78.

17. Marcus G. Singer in "On Duties to Oneself" provides an interesting argument against the possibility of talking, in any strict sense, of duties to oneself, and thus indirectly against duties not to commit suicide, pp. 202-205.

18. "Code of Medical Ethics of the American Medical Association," Sec. 4, pp. 2-3.

19. Owsei Temkin, "Medicine in 1847 — Continental Europe," in "One Hundred Years Ago: A Symposium Presented by the Johns Hopkins Institute of the History of Medicine," *Bulletin of the History of Medicine* 21 (1947): 475-476.

20. A. M. Lassek, *Human Dissection: Its Drama and Struggle* (Springfield: Charles C. Thomas, 1958). There have been a number of attempts, for example, to prohibit by law potentially harmful experimentation on fetuses, such as the law enacted by the state of Minnesota, Minn. Sess. Law ch. 562, § 145.42 (1973), and to prosecute physicians who engage in experimentation on fetal material. See Donald Day, "Fetal Study Stirs Grand Jury in Abortion Debate," *Hospital Tribune*, April 8, 1974, 1, 28.

21. Plato, *Laws* 720 c-d, *The Collected Dialogues of Plato*, ed. Edith Hamilton and Huntington Cairns, trans. A. E. Taylor (Princeton: Princeton University Press, 1963), pp. 1310-11.

SAMUEL GOROVITZ

Dealing With Dying

1. I want to consider some of the moral issues that arise in respect to medical treatment of the dying. In the attempt, I will seek some clarity about what dying is and who is considered as doing it, what medical treatment is and why the dying get it, and what moral problems are and how we can deal with them.

My concern is with those who are dying and with some of the circumstances surrounding them. Such persons, of course, are very much among the living. Still, I do need to focus some attention on the subject of death, since it is death that gives dying its special poignancy. Does it make sense to fear death, to seek to avoid it, and to lament it when it comes to others?

A death can occur too soon or too late. Further, there is the question of how it will come about. There are dyings that are slow and agonizing, and dyings that are gentle and graceful. It's the latter sort to which one aspires, but there is a substantial risk of being overtaken by froward circumstances. It seems reasonable that, given conditions that make death impending, one should want to exert some influence on the mode of dying. Just as one wants to be able to influence the major events that shape and constitute a life at earlier stages, one may want to avoid the indignity of having to witness and endure a final stage not as an efficacious agent, but merely a deteriorating object.

A death will come too soon if one has, as it approaches, aspirations and projects which engage one's interest and hence endow one's on-going life with value for one. As B. A. O. Williams has observed, "To want something . . . is to that extent to have a reason for resisting what excludes having that thing; and death certainly does that, for a very large range of things that one wants."[1] Thus it is reasonable for one to view one's future death as an evil so long as one is up to something one cares about with which it will interfere. That death is no evil to the dead does not entail that it is no evil to the living.

On the other hand, one's death comes too late if, lacking aspirations and projects that carry one forward, one's life drags on devoid of the point that only one's purposes could give it.

Thus there are two distinct respects in which one's dying can be an object of one's disapproval. One may do it in a bad way and one may do it at a bad time.

This sense of a well-timed death arises in part from a biographical sense of life — that is, of the life that each person leads. It is not grandiose for people to consider their lives as biographies in making. Every life *is* a biography in the making, even though most are of limited public interest and, at the hands of most biographers, not worth writing. This sense of one's life, moreover, can be overdone, as when one begins to act for the sake of the story, choosing what to do primarily on the basis of an aesthetic sense of what will make the best literary material.

Still, our aesthetic sense has a place here. In assessing a life about which we are reading, we may judge that the life, overall, was less happy or noble or valuable than it might otherwise have been, in virtue of having ended badly. And our sense of a bad ending is not merely based on simplistic considerations of whether there was pain in the dying or whether aspirations were left unfulfilled. Our sense of a bad ending involves our sense of the story as a whole. For Hemingway to die by his own hand in the face of physical deterioration seems fitting in a way in which other suicides may not be. One may quite reasonably desire that the story of one's life not be a tragic tale, and that it be a tale rich with character development, coherence of plot, and other literary virtues — including an ending that makes sense, both in mode and moment, in the context of what has gone before.

I believe this way of contemplating a life has an advantage: it helps us achieve a valuable detachment from our usual absorption in living. Such detachment is essential for our being able to take stock of our lives in order to exercise judgment about and reasoned influence on the shapes our lives take.

2. Ortega y Gasset claimed that "Life is of no consequence if a formidable eagerness to widen its frontiers does not stamp

within its confines."[2] For some of us, his observation strikes a responsive cord. Yet even if we accept such a criterion of having consequence as being applicable to our own lives, we must be wary of imposing it on others. There is really no telling what will make another person's life have consequence for him. That will depend on the sorts of projects and aspirations that he has. The more they differ from our own, the harder it will be for us to identify with that person, but such difficulty should not incline us to want to impose more familiar and hence more comfortable criteria of meaningfulness on other people's lives. It follows that our judgment about the ending of another person's life is one that cannot be well made in ignorance of some knowledge about the story of that life.

If we know enough about that story, we may see the final stage — the dying — as nothing to combat before the fact or lament after the fact, nor its mode appropriate to alter. The dying may be proceeding just as its subject would have it, given the constraints imposed by the physical and social worlds. It is thus possible for me to see the death and the dying of another as no evils for that person, and to refuse to lament them on that other's account — not from any insouciance, but from the conviction that there is nothing to lament. At the same time, I may with complete consistency sorely grieve my loss in the other's death — for my interest in another's life may be substantially different from his. For example, I may have a deep emotional dependence on a woman whose life, my dependence on it notwithstanding, holds no point or prospects for her. Or I may be the agent of a writer whose death is a good one in the context of her total life story, but which at the same time deals me a severe economic blow. Or I may be a physician attending a patient whose death, welcome and benign from the patient's point of view, aggravates my anxiety, erodes my ego, and sullies my statistics. But if I have no vested interest in the other's life, no reason for valuing its continuation, and if its continuation has no value for that other, then it is hard to see why its continuation should be perceived as having any value at all. If we begin with the assumption that it must have value, it may be of use to become clear about whose purposes and needs give rise to that assumption.

I am not suggesting that anyone's dying should be taken lightly. On the contrary, I am saying that if we take a person's dying seriously — as seriously as we would take a person's education, marriage, or career — then we must consider it as that person's own, unique dying, the final stage of a particular life. To consider it thus is to require of ourselves that we see it in the context of the story of that life, and not merely as one more instance of a general evil. It is far easier, of course, simply to dig in on the side of life, and repel the rebarbative reaper however we can.

But do we clearly understand just what the reaper represents? What constitutes death is not a fact to discover, but a decision to make. We easily identify clear cases of life — such as a person actively engaged in some familiar enterprise, and of death — such as the decaying remains of a former person. In between, we can find hard cases. It was once thought that what, if anything, was hard about cases at the border was the task of discovering whether, as a matter of empirical fact, the vital forces or substances had departed quite yet, or merely seemed to have. Now we can know what is physiologically true of a patient without knowing whether or not to call that patient dead. When we seek a definition of death to help resolve the issue, we find that no definition is defensible except as tested against an independent judgment about whether or not we wish to classify people in such circumstances as dead or alive. So we cannot look to definitions to decide the case; we must decide the case as part of the process of fashioning and testing the definition. The kind of case that is often cited to illustrate the point is that of the patient with severe, irreversible damage to the neocortex, who sustains enough brain-stem function to maintain spontaneous circulatory and respiratory activity indefinitely in total absence of consciousness or any prospect of consciousness. What shall we decide of such a case?

The arguments that surround the issue are well known, and I will not rehearse them. I will emphasize one aspect of the debate that is apposite. The definition of death that we endorse reflects our reasons for valuing life. If we hold, as I would hold, that it is only experiences that have intrinsic value, then it is plain why life is precious. Life is the precondition of experience, and hence is a *sine qua non* of all that has value. But this view, while accounting for the preciousness of life, does so in a way that bases that preciousness on the connection between life, which has instrumental value, and the experience it makes possible, which alone can have intrinsic value. Where there is not experience or prospect of experience, such life as is present loses its lustre. In the case at issue, we may say that the biologically viable organism, devoid irreversibly of sentience, has life that is no longer of value and that we may thus abandon with impunity. And the device by which we abandon life that has no value may be to declare death. Thus a criterion of death that is based on evidence of neocortical function may reflect our prior judgment that such life as can be sustained without it and the experience for which it is apparently essential is life devoid of value, and hence a sort of death.

But if we hold, as some do, that life itself has intrinsic value, then the question of sentience does not arise. The irrevocably comatose are nonetheless alive for their lack of sentience, and their lives, having the value that inheres in all human life, must be sustained. No definition or criterion in terms of neocortical activity will do. Our patient is alive after all, and thus qualifies for care.

Our conceptions of value are thus intertwined with our criteria of classification. As medical intervention more subtly, sensitively, and selectively separates the complex farrago of functions that constitute a fully living person, we see a continuum of states emerging that ranges from the clearly living to the clearly dead through those who are alive in some ways and dead in others. How we want to relate to the mixed and marginal cases determines what we take death to be, and the moral and conceptual issues are not separable.

The search for an operational definition of death is, of course, motivated in large measure by the desire to fashion guidelines for the resolution of clinical quandaries. Which definition of death is adopted can have immediate behavioral consequences, sometimes of a dramatic sort. Either the kidney is made available in time for the life-saving transplantation or it is not. Either the intravenous feeding continues and the patient is kept in a bed, or it stops and the corpse is put in a coffin. Either the family lingers on in an indeterminate agony of resignation beyond hope or hope beyond reason, or the family shifts to the patterns of behavior appropriate to mourning their loss. And so on. It is no wonder a palatable definition of death is earnestly sought.

3. Lost in the search is the fact that we also classify people, at various times and in various ways during their lives, as dying. Little attention has been paid to what it means to speak of someone as dying, yet this too has behavioral consequences. They are not the decisive and dramatic consequences associated with disputes over definitions of death. Yet, in subtler ways, how we think of what dying is affects how we treat and relate to people. Let us therefore shift the focus from death to dying.

Life in full flower is an on-going actualization of possibilities. Even Oblomov, to whom action was anathema, was carried forward from one moment to the next by deliberations about the possibilities before him, and the constant reaffirmation of his indecisiveness became for him a mode of acting that gave his life its special stamp.[3] Dying closes off possibilities. Human relationships consist in a shared actualizing of possibilities available for choice. Dying thus transforms relationships, replacing the sense of future that nourishes them with a sense of ending that tends to impoverish them. So it matters a great deal whether or not one is classified as dying.

Stalin is reputed to have replied to inquiry about a rumored fatal illness, "Of course I am dying. I have been since the day I was born." We are all dying in this sense, synonymous with 'mortal', that makes no distinctions among us. But as Bishop Butler distinguished the selfish from the selfish, we must distinguish the dying from the dying — by seeking an account of 'dying' that captures the sense of that term that is associated with impending death as opposed to eventual death.[4] Again, we can readily identify clear cases. Ivan Ilych on his penultimate day is dying;[5] Hans Castorp, as his journey to the mountains begins, is not.[6] In between, it is a matter of some dispute.

What are the conditions under which it is correct to say of someone that he is dying? We can approach the question by reminding ourselves of what sorts of circumstances lead us to think of someone as dying. The paradigmatic cases in fashionable forums on fatality seem to be a terminally ill adult, diagnosed as having a short but indeterminate life expectancy, whose physician isn't sure about what to say, and a pain-wracked or insensate patient at the brink of death, whose physician isn't sure about how or whether to intervene. The dying, however, are not necessarily aged or diseased; they include the injured, the young, and perhaps those whose plight is more a function of circumstances than of health, such as trapped and isolated miners, astronauts, and divers. Is there anything they all have in common?

As a first approximation to an analysis, I suggest that a person can correctly be said to be dying if three conditions are satisfied. These conditions are:

Condition 1.   A. The person has a generally irreversible illness known to lead to death, *or*

B. The person is inextricably in circumstances known to lead to death, *or*

C. The person exhibits deterioration of a sort known to lead to death.

Condition 2.   There is strong reason to believe that the person will die of that illness, circumstance, or deterioration.

Condition 3.   The death is likely to occur soon.

The first condition has three parts to correspond to three different kinds of cases. A covers the typical fatally ill person, such as one with severe leukemia. B covers the physiologically sound person in fatal circumstances, such as the astronaut cut adrift in space with inadequate oxygen. C covers the patient who, lacking an identifiable illness, has symptoms that preclude survival — such as severe and accelerating loss of weight and strength, accompanied by soaring fever, depressed respiration, etc.

Condition 2 is necessary to rule out cases that trivially satisfy 1. For example, a person over 30 is inextricably in circumstances known to lead to death.[7] But there is no strong reason to believe that the cause of death will be those circumstances, directly or indirectly, so we cannot consider such a person to be dying, even though 1B is trivially satisfied. Condition 3 is needed to distinguish between someone simply at substantial risk, such as one with a chronic weak heart, from one actually in the process of dying. A person with an extremely bad heart might satisfy conditions 1 and 2, yet not be dying because no fatal process of change is under way — no worsening of condition or circumstances is taking place. But then condition 3 is not satisfied, for only a process of worsening can justify the judgment that the death will occur soon. In sum, that person is dying who has a generally irreversible illness or pattern of deterioration, or is inextricably in circumstances, known to lead to and cause death soon.

Each condition, of course, could use substantial further explication, and probably requires further refinement. For example, condition 2 refers to a person's dying "of" the illness, circumstance or deterioration in virtue of which he is said to be dying. But many patients, weakened by one illness, die of a second induced by the first. Thus, the cancer patient may succumb in the end to pneumonia, which he would not have contracted but for the cancer. One might want to hold that although the cancer led to the death, the patient did not die *of* the cancer. Condition 2 must be interpreted to accommodate such cases.

But it does not matter at all whether this account is correct in detail. What is important is only that the correct account will be essentially like this one in certain respects. Any explication of the above conditions would likely focus on such notions as those of strong reasons, of dying soon, of what is generally irreversible or inextricable. The conditions depend essentially on these elusive notions, and, if I am right, any correct analysis of dying will share that dependency.

What these notions have in common is their judgmental quality. What counts as dying soon can never be measured by an EEG; we decide what counts as a sufficiently imminent death to qualify one as dying in part on the basis of how we want to treat and relate to people in various circumstances. We decide what are inextricable circumstances in part on the basis of what our priorities are for allocating the resources available to us. And so on. Thus we decide who the dying are not merely on the basis of discoverable medical fact, but also on the basis of value-laden judgments that are presupposed by our conceptions of what it is to be dying.

It is commonly assumed, at least implicitly, that the definitional problems concern death, and that since dying is simply approaching death, what counts as dying will be determined once it is resolved what is to count as death. I have argued that this is simply not so — that even given agreement about what constitutes death, our taxonomy is value-laden.

4.   Those who are judged to be dying are often in, or about to be in, the hands of providers of medical treatment. Before confronting directly the moral issues that arise in connection with medical treatment of the dying, however, we should note the variety of ways in which physicians and their associates can relate to dying persons.

The first relationship is diagnostic; primarily the physician is the one who classifies a patient as dying. If the patient's condition is bad enough, the physician may classify him instead as already having died, in which case the function is one of pronouncement and certification, rather than of diagnosis or treatment. If the patient is diagnosed as dying, the most common relationship between the physician and the patient is that of medical intervention aimed at forestalling death — at holding it at bay for as long as possible. Sometimes, however, the physician relinquishes his resistance and acquiesces in the arrival of death, shifting his focus from the patient's survival to the patient's physical comfort. The physician may even facilitate the ending, for example, by withdrawing or withholding certain treatments, or by making the means of suicide available. In extreme cases, the physician may go beyond facilitating death, actively intervening to terminate the life in his care.

These functions — judging, forestalling, facilitating, and terminating — are the most obvious medical functions in relation to dying. But the proper responsibilities and objectives of medicine include other functions. The stunningly increased efficacy of medical intervention for forestalling death seems to have overshadowed the function of dealing supportively with the living problems of the dying patient. It is one benefit of the recent popularity of death as a topic that some redress of this imbalance seems to be under way.[8] The kind of work exemplified by the efforts of Dr. Kübler-Ross or at St. Christopher's Hospice in London demonstrates the value of accepting dying patients for what they are, and striving to serve their needs.[9] Finally, the physician bears a responsibility for dealing with those problems of survivors that relate to the dying and death of others — of attending to the aftermath of death. Let us consider each of the six functions briefly in turn.

I have argued that the judgmental function is not simply a matter of the application of scientific or medical expertise, but depends on evaluative assumptions that different persons might not share. A patient, assuming he knows the medical facts that are true of him, might consider himself to be dying, as judged from the perspective of his life story and the values that infuse it; his physician, perhaps unaware of the patient's aspirations and priorities for resource allocation, may not perceive the patient as dying. Insofar as the "dying" label changes one's sense of the possibilities or influences the way others perceive and relate to one, the difference in judgment between the physician and the patient can underlie a difference about how it is appropriate to treat the patient. Of course, insofar as the patient is unable, in virtue of ignorance of the medical facts or for other reasons, to make an informed judgment on the issue, his ability to participate autonomously in decisions about his treatment is curtailed.

The moral problems associated with forestalling death are more obvious. The usual list includes: the question of the justifiability of using extended exotic therapies to forestall the death of a patient whose prospects for life are tenebrous at best; the question of the extent to which and ways in which it is justifiable to incorporate economic considerations into decisions about whether, how, and for how long to attempt to forestall death; and the question of the extent to which others than the dying have obligations to participate in the effort to forestall death, e.g., by donating blood or a kidney. There are other questions as well. Pervading them all is the more fundamental question of whether death is always an evil to be combatted, or whether under some conditions a more accepting posture is appropriate. The debates about suicide, euthanasia, and death with dignity begin at this point.

Facilitating death seems at first, to be an intermediate relationship somewhere between accepting death and causing it. Applying the concept, however, is not always easy. Recall the famous case at Johns Hopkins Hospital of the Down's Syndrome baby with duodenal atresia, whose life could have been saved by surgery had the parents allowed it, but who died instead after many days in the hospital without food or medical treatment.[10] In the debate that has followed public disclosure of that case, some have argued that the hospital personnel simply let the baby die. Others hold that the baby was killed, no less than had it been injected with potassium chloride — though perhaps less mercifully. If facilitating death lies between letting it happen and causing it, it is hard to see how the notion can clarify the case at hand.

If a normal child with a curable infection dies because the antibiotic that defeats the infection was withheld either inadvertently or deliberately, we are inclined to view that withholding as having culpably caused the death. If the child is instead a neonatal monster, we are more inclined to see the withholding as a simple non-interference with benign natural processes. If the patient is in the late stages of an excruciating terminal illness, the decision not to treat may be viewed as facilitating the imminent death, as might the intended administration of a dosage of analgesic that suppresses respiration in a way that invites infection.

Philosophers are fond of arguing for the non-existence of what others take for granted. Sometimes such arguments strike the plain man as fantasy. But the philosopher's skepticism can not always be easily dismissed. Actors in the dramas that constitute much of modern medicine often do accept as legitimate, clear, and important the ostensible distinctions among killing, facilitating death, and letting die. Thus, the Euthanasia Society argues for passive euthanasia — an intended allowing to die under certain circumstances, while explicitly not advocating active euthanasia — the intentional intervention to terminate life.[11] And troubled physicians sometimes find solace in the thought that whereas they could never be a party to deliberate termination of life, a humane acceptance of the approach of death requires that they let some patients die by refraining from providing or even imposing treatment that is available. But other physicians, perhaps somewhat more reflective, are less comfortable with these distinctions.

Here, the philosopher's skepticism may find its mark. The arguments are strong that acts of omission are as significant causally and morally as their more visible counterparts, the acts of commission.[12] If I can prevent your death by giving you the antidote to a poison you have inadvertently taken, it is hard to see how my deliberate refraining from doing so can be distinguished morally from my giving you poison in the first place. But unless some such distinction can be made out, the physician who *allows* a patient to die, in peace and dignity or in any other way, when the means of forestalling death were available, is indulging himself in a deception — comforting, perhaps, but a deception still — when he believes his behavior is morally different from active euthanasia.

Some people take the difficulty of distinguishing among allowing, facilitating, and causing death to constitute a part of the argument in favor of making every effort to forestall death. Others use the same point in support of active euthanasia. Thus the issues surrounding the termination of life are inseparable from those surrounding allowing or facilitating death.

The function of caring supportively for the dying patient raises different kinds of concerns. Nobody likes to invest in a losing proposition, and dying persons are losing propositions from many points of view. Emotional capital is limited, for health-care providers as well as everyone else. There seems to be no long term payoff from investing it in dying strangers. Caring for people diminishes the extent to which they are strangers. Further, our emotions, widely known to prompt our actions, also follow our actions. Thus we tend to care *about* those we take care *of*. (The ambiguity of 'caring for' may be more than coincidence.)[13] It is thus no surprise that once a person is accepted as dying, the inclination to care for that person declines markedly. The induration faced by dying persons in hospitals is particularly well reported of late; it is in hospitals most of all that dying is an affront to one's hosts, and hence is socially unacceptable behavior.

The values reflected by this familiar pattern of withdrawal from the dying are, I think, primarily utilitarian and specifically self-protective. Dying persons are nonetheless persons for their dying, and their need to sustain satisfying relationships with other persons is nonetheless intense for their circumstances being discomforting. For most of us, our patterns of relating to others are primarily predicated on the existence of future-oriented, on-going possibilities. To the extent that the dying person faces an attenuated future, those patterns of relating to people seem awkward, disingenuous, or even impossible. Yet a respect for the present needs of dying persons demands the fashioning of patterns of relating to them on terms that make sense for them. That requires going beyond the treatment of their pain and of their bodies. It requires at times the courage to join with them in an acknowledgment of their plight, legitimizing and participating in their efforts to come to terms with that plight.

Once a patient has died, attending to the aftermath frequently involves a physician, almost as an automatic consequence of his role as the one who certifies death and reports it to survivors. Once the death certificate is signed, the sedatives commonly follow close behind. Immediate reactions of shock, grief, relief, guilt, and all the rest that are bound up with confronting the death of someone close, are obvious and become the focus of medical care. Yet here we see an ironic reversal. The focus of attention on the dying person tends to be on the body — the physical organism with respect to which the physician has a repertoire of techniques of intervention. The emotional needs of the dying person are slighted, and thus we note the present campaign to reestablish an awareness of the living humanity of persons approaching death. Yet as soon as one turns from the dying patient to the survivors, psychological sensitivity reasserts itself, almost as if, no longer repressed by the minatory prospect of dealing with death, it is relieved at the chance to face less intimidating problems like grief or shock. Yet just as dying persons have minds as well as bodies, survivors have bodies as well as minds, and their bodies are placed in greater jeopardy by the stress of their loss.

The mortality rate for survivors of a death is markedly greater than for populations otherwise similar.[14] This effect can be seen both in humans and in some animal species. Creatures do die of grief and other stressful emotions that often accompany bereavement. Thus it is statistically true that the physical well being of the survivors of a death is eroded by that death. In a given case, of course, this effect may be wholly lacking; the merry widow's dalliance may begin to the strains of the dirge. The extent to which a given survivor's health is undermined by the death will depend in part on the role the deceased had played in the survivor's life. Knowing something of the story of that life thus may be an essential part of being able to attend responsibly to the aftermath of the death. In the days of the family physician, such familiarity with the special circumstances of survivors was more to be expected. Now, the deceased's oncologist, for example, may play a minor role in meeting the survivor's needs, and the survivor's own medical care may be in the hands of disparate specialists, an impersonal clinic, or, in the absence of symptoms at the time of the death, in no hands at all. Thus, certain aspects of attending to the aftermath of a death may get scant consideration, in part in consequence of the structure of modern health care delivery.

5.   We have taken a brief look at a sampling of morally significant problems that arise as physicians deal with dying. It is time for some observations about moral problems in general. They are problems of decision — of deciding which among a number of available actions is the right one to perform. Further, they involve conflict in the sense that there are reasons present in favor of at least two different and incompatible choices. Finally, the choices influence people in ways about which they care. Moral problems that gain substantial attention generate a strong sense of the possibility of serious error, and that sense in turn generates anxiety. In debates about abortion, euthanasia, and suicide,

as well as in those about sexual morality, modes of governance, and military undertakings, partisans project an air of the profound and the tragic. Not only is moral error possible, but the consequences of making it are severe. The basic challenge is thus to avoid error, and the ambivalence and uncertainty that pervade the context of decision make the challenge a difficult one.

Moral guidelines, if they are to be of use in such circumstances, must help us to distinguish among the available choices of action. It is no benefit to admonish an agent to do what he cannot avoid, or to do what is not possible. Significant guidance is that favoring what we can, but might not, choose to do. Moral rules, moreover, like the general moral principles that support them, must accurately reflect values we hold. But the most obvious traditional moral rules are inadequate for the resolution of moral conflicts. We may agree that killing people is wrong, yet almost no one seriously holds the view that the rule always provides the morally optimal judgment. Instead, we allow exceptions, such as self-defense, defense of family, or military excursions under certain arguable circumstances. For some, even conviction of certain crimes warrants termination of life, and for some, certain medical circumstances justify killing. The moral rule prohibiting killing applies most clearly where we need it least. We are not in conflict over the justifiability, for example, of shooting octogenarian pensioners for sport. The cases that constitute problems, such as those involving reasoned suicide or requested euthanasia, are precisely those where the applicability of the rule is in question, thus the rule cannot resolve such disputes for us. Since moral problems are in general of this character, there is no prospect of solving them by recourse to rules like that proscribing killing.

Some moral philosophers have seen their task as that of finding or fashioning a fundamental principle or set of principles that will capture our moral convictions, applying clearly to the uncontroversial cases and enabling us to resolve the controversial ones. None has succeeded, however. The task is difficult perhaps to the point of intractability, because our moral convictions are complex and inconsistent, at least against the backdrop of the real world. Thus we do value the prolongation of life and we do value relief from suffering, yet the workings of the world sometimes preclude our achieving both. Since we want both but cannot have both, we face the kind of conflict that generates moral dilemma and, hence, moral philosophy.

If it were possible to confirm a true moral theory of the kind that some have sought, we might then derive from it specific moral rules that would constitute a definitive set of guidelines for the resolution of moral problems that arise in dealing with dying patients. No such confirmation seems possible. Even those who accept a sweeping moral perspective, such as are provided by religious orthodoxies that advocate specific substantive positions about moral issues in medicine, frequently find themselves in conflict over particular cases.

The difficulty of solving specific moral problems without a generally accepted and complete theory of morality, combined with the apparent unavailability of any such theory, leads to skepticism about whether moral philosophy can shed any useful light on the problems faced in clinical practice.[15] In its most extreme form, such skepticism may yield the view that individual judgment and individual conscience, in all their diversity, are the only resources available for the resolution of the hard cases. I do not believe such radical skepticism is warranted. A full response to it is not possible here. However, I will try to temper it by ending with a few more thoughts about clinical practice.

I have said that moral dilemmas challenge us to avoid making errors in choosing among possible courses of action. But it is naive to think of moral error as limited simply to the selection of the wrong alternative, as if one's life as a moral agent is an on-going multiple-choice exam. Another sort of moral error, perhaps more significant, involves the *ways* in which the choices, for better or worse, are made. The issue is one of moral integrity, the ingredients of which are not wholly arcane. They include the requirement that one act in any given situation with concern, conscientiousness, and courage in proportion to the gravity of that situation. The irreversibility of death gives those situations that involve it a reverberating gravity. Thus, in dealing with dying, one faces strict standards if moral integrity is to be maintained. Conscientiousness in such situations involves acknowledging the humanity of dying persons — that is, acknowledging that the death that is approaching can only be judged in the context of the story of the life that it will end, and that context involves the patient's beliefs and attitudes as much as his physiological characteristics. The conscientious physician will have the courage to face his own feelings about death, the honesty to distinguish between his own interest in the patient's life and the patient's interest in that life, and the concern to invest the requisite time and effort to understand enough of the story of that life to make decisions in an informed way.[16] Even satisfying such conditions of conscientiousness, the physician dealing with a dying patient can not be certain that his (the physician's) actions fully respect the values that he would endorse on reflection; more likely he will know regret from time to time. Accepting one's own moral missteps, however — acknowledging and learning from them without arrogance or defeatism — is also an aspect of moral integrity.

The physician, then, even without standards of morality that can conclusively resolve all his dilemmas, can still adopt as a morally compelling objective the goal of acting always with as much moral integrity as he can muster. He can still seek to maximize his patient's autonomy with respect to the mode and conditions of death, knowing that doing so requires that the physician accept and provide information that is discomforting for him to acknowledge openly. He can never wholly dispel anguish, but he need not despair. Instead of striving always to maximize life, he can pursue the nobler and more arduous task of aiding his dying patients to write as fitting a final chapter as circumstances will allow to the stories of their lives.

NOTES

I am indebted at many points throughout this paper to Bernard Williams, Robert Veatch, Joseph Margolis, and William Ruddick for ideas that arose in lectures and conversations at the Moral Problems in Medicine Institute sponsored by the Council for Philosophical Studies in 1974, with the support of the Rockefeller Brothers Fund. I have also benefited from conversations on an earlier draft from Ruth Macklin and Lawrence Stern. Their agreement with my views should not be presumed, however.

1. B. Williams, "The Makropulos Case: Reflections on the Tedium of Immortality" in *Problems of the Self* (New York: Cambridge University Press, 1973), p. 85.

2. Ortega y Gasset, "The Dehumanization of Art" in *A Modern Book of Esthetics*, ed. M. Rader, 3rd edn. (New York: Holt, Rinehart and Winston, 1960), p. 419.

3. I. Goncharov, *Oblomov*.

4. The discussion appears in Butler's eleventh sermon, reprinted as Sermon IV in J. Butler *Five Sermons* (Indianapolis: Bobbs-Merrill, 1950).

5. L. Tolstoy, *The Death of Ivan Ilych*.

6. T. Mann, *The Magic Mountain*.

7. The age is arbitrary; any number that is not too high will do.

8. Cf., for example, the bibliography in D. Hendin, *Death as a Fact of Life* (New York: Norton, 1973), pp. 229-41, and the *Bibliography of Society, Ethics and the Life Sciences,* 1974, pp. 68-77.

9. E. Kübler-Ross, *On Death and Dying* (New York: Macmillan Co., 1969), and R. Neale, "A Place of Live and a Place to Die," *The Hastings Center Report* 2, No. 2, June 1972, pp. 12-14.

10. This case is re-enacted in *Who Should Survive,* a 24 minute film produced by the Joseph R. Kennedy, Jr. Foundation and distributed by the Joseph P. Kennedy Jr. Foundation Film Servie, 999 Asylum Avenue, Hartford, Conn.

11. Cf., for example, the argument presented in *The Right to Die,* a 60 minute documentary film produced by ABC News and distributed by MacMillan Films, Inc., Mt. Vernon, N.Y.

12. Cf., for example, J. J. Thomson, "Killing, Letting Die, and the Trolly Problem," *The Monist,* 59 (1976): 204-17.

13. Cf. Plato's *Euthyphro*.

14. W. Rees, and S. Lutkins, "Mortality of Bereavement," *British Medical Journal,* October 1967.

15. Cf., A MacIntyre, "How Virtues Become Vices," and S. Gorovitz, "Moral Philosophy and Medical Perplexity," in *Explanation and Evaluation in the Biomedical Sciences,* ed. T. Engelhardt, Jr., and S. Spicker, (Dordrecht: D. Reidel, 1975).

16. C. Whal, "The Fear of Death" *Bulletin of the Menninger Clinic,* 22, 1958.

JAMES F. TOOLE, M.D. L.L.B.

The Concept of Brain Death
as Viewed by a Neurologist

In 1927, Dr. Francis W. Peabody began his famous series of talks to Harvard medical students on "The Care of the Patient" with this remark: "The most common criticism made at present by older practitioners is that young graduates have been taught a great deal about the mechanism of disease, but very little about the practice of medicine — or, to put it more bluntly, they are too 'scientific' and do not know how to take care of patients." [1] He criticized the impersonal atmosphere of hospitals where diseases, not people, are treated and where any distress in the family caused by the illness is ignored. Therefore, Dr. Peabody called upon physicians to consider the whole patient — his disease, his personality, his place in society, and his relationship with his family and to prescribe his treatment accordingly.

Almost 50 years later the situation is, if anything, worse not better, and the need for an awareness of the total patient is nowhere greater than among neurologists, whose responsibility it is to diagnose and treat diseases of the brain, which, many believe, makes a body into a human being. Despite this need, neurologists have traditionally been more attracted to scientific appraisal of a disease process than to management of the patient and his family.

But what does this have to do with the concept of brain death as viewed by a neurologist? Just this — humanism was expunged from neurology when the founders of my discipline opted for the scientific approach. As a consequence, we are now faced with a situation in which the very physicians who are the most knowledgeable about the field of brain death are the ones least likely to approach the problem with a well-rounded viewpoint. Obviously there are many exceptions to this generalization, of which Charles D. Aring, Daniel Silverman, and the late Lord Russell Brain are but three.[2]

Consequently, it is not surprising that the concept of brain death did not emanate, as one might have suspected, from neurologists or neurosurgeons but from an anesthesiologist, Henry Beecher,[3] whose perspective was the Intensive Care Unit where respirators maintained "life" long after brain function had ceased. He chaired the ad hoc committee of Harvard Medical School that legitimatized what many had recognized as a problem but few were doing anything about. The committee's report[4] served as the stimulus for formalizing the concept of brain death.

Brain Death Criteria

Before the 1968 Harvard report, the courts in this country generally supported the traditional concept that death occurred when there was "a total stoppage of the circulation of the blood, and a cessation of the animal and vital functions consequent thereto such as respiration and pulsation, etc."[5] The Harvard group believed that such a definition was inadequate in view of modern advancements in medicine, e.g., the ability to sustain life through the use of supportive measures even when a patient's brain is irreversibly damaged. Therefore, they proposed irreversible coma as a new definition of death and suggested that the following criteria be met to establish this diagnosis: unreceptivity or unresponsivity to external stimuli, no spontaneous muscular movements or respiration, no reflexes, and an isoelectric electroencephalogram. In addition, they recommended repeating all tests after 24 hours and cautioned that test results must be verified as not being caused by hypothermia or central nervous system depressants, such as barbiturates.[6]

Although the term 'brain death' is generally used to refer to these new criteria, the above definition makes it clear that they "assess not only higher brain functions but brainstem and spinal cord activity"[7] and the respiratory nerves and muscles as well. The common terminology 'brain death' is, therefore, somewhat misleading.

Legislation

As of late 1974 only three states — Kansas, Maryland, and Virginia — had enacted statutes that legalize new brain death criteria for determining the time of death.[8] The Kansas and Maryland statutes stipulate that death occurs when there is an "absence of spontaneous respiratory and cardiac functions" or an "absence of spontaneous brain function."[9] Neither requires a consulting physician to corroborate the determination of brain death. The Virginia statute defines death according to the same two criteria; however, it requires the attendance of a consulting physician who must be a neurologist, a neurosurgeon, or an electroencephalographer.[10] The Kansas statute has been widely criticized as giving rise to "the misconception that there are two separate phenomena of death."[11] Actually, all three statutes could be critized on this score. Furthermore, critics believe that Kansas statute was enacted for the benefit of the transplant surgeon and was intended to facilitate organ transplantation rather than to establish uniform criteria for determining death.[12]

Professional Acceptance

While physicians generally endorse this new concept of death,[13] the American Medical Association has discouraged the enactment of legislation to legalize the new criteria.[14] Dr. Beecher, Chairman of the Harvard committee, recommends that new legislation be postponed until the medical profession can further clarify its definition of death. He fears the codification of present standards will prohibit the introduction of new ones.[15] The difficulties of legislating criteria are well stated by Capron:

> The legislative alternative . . . has a number of drawbacks. . . . A statute "defining" death may be badly drafted. It may be either too general or too specific, or it may be so poorly worded that it will leave physicians or laymen unsure of its intent. There is also the danger that the statutory language might seem to preclude further refinements that expanding medical knowledge would introduce into the tests and procedures for determining death.[16]

Public Acceptance

Surprisingly, the concept of brain death has been embraced more quickly by the public than by the medical profession. Many people have signed a document called "The Living Will," which requests that no life lengthening measures be used if they are terminally ill. Although not legally binding, the "will" indicates the person's wish that when "there is no reasonable expectation of my recovery from physical or mental disability, . . . I be allowed to die and not be kept alive by artificial means or 'heroic measures.' "[17] The public seems to recognize what neurologists have generally believed, that the essence of humanity is mind. Because a dead brain contains no mind, remaining life is no longer human and can be extinguished without violation of ethical codes.

The attitude of the public has been profoundly affected by the ability of modern medicine to prolong life artificially far beyond its natural limits. Many people fear such an unnatural end to their lives. One personal statement is revealing:

> The average duration of life . . . has increased greatly in the past half century. This change is usually referred to as an unmixed blessing. But is it? Where I question its value is in the prolongation of helpless old age.
>
> My father and mother died on the farm at about sixty. Until their last illnesses, they were active and vigorous. . . . All of their brothers and sisters went to the city. . . . In their protected environments, they have gone on living, until their average age is eighty. One is blind, one is terribly crippled with rheumatism, the keen mind of another is entirely faded. . . .
>
> They still say to me, "If only your mother could have led an easier life, she might be with us still." But there has never been a question in my mind that her fate was kinder.
>
> My friends and I feel that after mature consideration, . . . one should be allowed to drink the hemlock in some dignified and simple way.[18]

But there are those who have the opposite reaction to death. Recently, a 39-year-old physician died of cancer of the bowel, but before his death he made a series of videotapes concerning his feelings about dying. This doctor did not want to die and desperately struggled to prolong his life as long as possible despite extreme pain and physical deterioration. His "doctors agreed that he [had] pushed them to decisions they would not otherwise have made. Though some doctors said [the patient's] life [had] been unnecessarily prolonged . . . , his widow insisted that every day he [managed] to stay alive was of great value to him."[19] Perhaps his relative youth was a crucial factor in his difficulty in accepting death.

Capron notes some disquiet among the public over "the prospect of physicians agreeing amongst themselves to change the rules by which life is measured"[20] without consulting with the public at large. "The idea of death is at least partly a philosophical question. . . . Physicians qua physicians are not expert on these philosophical questions, nor are they expert on the question of which physiological functions decisively identify a 'living, human organism.' "[21] Therefore, Capron and others [22] advocate involving the public in these extra-medical decisions.

A NEUROLOGIST'S VIEWPOINT

To present a neurologist's perspective on the brain death concept, I will first consider the criteria for the diagnosis of brain death, second, mention some of the possible legal consequences and moral dilemmas posed by this redefinition of death, and, third, discuss different philosophies of treatment among medical staff.

Application of Brain Death Criteria

With regard to the diagnosis of brain death, it is apparent that physicians conversant with neurological diagnosis can with a high degree of certainty make this diagnosis on clinical grounds alone. The distinction should be stressed, however, that only a physician with more than the usual competence in neurology can assess a patient's condition to determine death by these criteria. Even the electroencephalographer is competent only to pass on the interpretation of the brain waves because he does not examine the patient.

The three major categories of patients in whom brain death is likely to precede death of the other parts of the body are

1. Those with cranial trauma,

2. Those with primary intracranial catastrophe, such as hemorrhage, and
3. Those who do not recover consciousness after cardiopulmonary resuscitation or following surgery.

In these groups of patients the prolonged absence of all voluntary and reflex activity strongly suggests a diagnosis of brain death if poisoning by anesthetics or undue cooling of the body can be ruled out. We can determine precisely the loss of brainstem functions such as the pupillary responses to light, labyrinthine response to ice-water caloric stimulation, oculo cardiac reflex, and spontaneous respiration. In addition, we can assess the loss of spinal cord function by the absence of stretch reflexes. If poisoning and hypothermia are not the cause and if this state persists for 24 hours, one can be virtually certain that brainstem and spinal cord death has occurred. It is still conceivable, however, that the cerebrum survives, and for this reason, as well as for the objective evidence that it provides, verifying electrocerebral silence on two electroencephalograms spaced two hours apart according to the technical criteria for recording recommended by the American EEG Society seems prudent.[23]

Some investigators have reported a return of activity in the electroencephalogram (EEG) after a period of electrocerebral silence. In two case reports, involving an infant and a child, EEG's repeated after 24 hours changed from silence to activity.[24] Repetition of the EEG would provide an adequate safeguard against this possibility.

The requirement of concurrence by an electroencephalographer shifts some of the decision-making burden from the bedside clinician to the electroencephalographer. The latter sits in the silence of his laboratory — a situation which electroencephalographers find quite uncomfortable for they recognize the subjective element in their interpretations.[25] They are unsettled by such questions as whether true electrocerebral silence has developed, or whether occasional deviations from the baseline are the result of artifact in the recording situation or cerebral rhythms. However, to differentiate brain waves from interfering noise, a number of approaches are available, such as the use of a digital computer to subtract out electrocardiogram sounds, the use of the isopotential line of the EEG, and the application of spectral analysis.

Another problem that haunts electroencephalographers is the fact that even in the isopotential EEG, prominent auditory-evoked potentials can often be elicited. Obviously these would not occur if there were not viable brain tissue.

Furthermore, scalp recordings may not be sufficiently sensitive to pick up rhythms of very low potential, and therefore some have suggested that corticograms or depth recordings be obtained. Dr. Reginald Bickford has devised an integrator that plots a continuous record of the voltage output of the brain calibrated in microvolts per minute.[26] This integrator has the advantages of being completely objective and of giving a continuous record so that the possibility of interpretation error is largely eliminated.

Another index of brain death, absence of blood flow through the organ, can be measured in a variety of ways, the simplest being the use of radioisotopic techniques for assessment of brain circulation and cerebral blood flow.[27] Alternatively, angiography of the carotid circulation showing nonfilling of the intracranial arteries can be used.[28] Where cerebral blood flow can be demonstrated to have ceased despite a normal systemic arterial blood pressure, brain survival is impossible, but the fallacy in these techniques is that they do not assess possible vertebrobasilar flow.

Echoencephalography for presence or absence of brain pulsation is another measure of brain circulation. In its absence, cerebral flow is probably nil in most cases.[29]

Other possible means for assessing the viability of the brain that have not been fully explored are tests for brain metabolism, such as oxygen consumption and CO_2 production, or the elaboration of products of metabolism or neurohumors.

Given time and interest, the skilled clinician, with the aid of electroencephalography and techniques for assessing cerebral circulation, will be able to diagnose the presence or absence of brain death with certainty.

Of course, an exceptional case does occur occasionally in which a person who has been declared dead spontaneously starts breathing again. Sometimes science cannot explain such recoveries. Recently, a young girl suffered severe brain injuries in an automobile accident. Six days later she "died," having no respiration, movement, or reflexes. However, during preparation for surgery to remove her kidneys for transplantation, she began to breathe again spontaneously. The press report speculates that "something in preparation for the transplant procedure — removal and reapplication of oxygen pumping equipment, stimulants injected to keep the kidneys functioning, physical movement of her body — could have jarred her back to life."[30]

Such cases are quite rare and do not deter from the high probability of ascertaining true death, but they have an enormous shock value to the public.

Legal Consequences and Moral Dilemmas

Sympathetic and biased as I am to the need for and the reasons underlying this movement for redefinition, I have long been gnawed by questions about the brain death concept and the possibility of some unpleasant consequences.[31]

As a neurologist, it is my profession to care for patients, segments of whose brains have been destroyed and whose function is lost forever, and herein lies the problem. How much brain must be destroyed before mind is lost permanently? Currently the problem is theoretical because total loss of all brain function, not only mind, is required before declaring a person dead because of brain death, but I predict that in the future this will change.

The brain is a collection of about 60 billion cells, called neurons, which interconnect to form the most complicated object in the universe. Groups of neurons with similar functions form cooperating centers and it is these centers that keep us conscious, control our respirations, and store our memories. Therefore, I ask, must every one of the sixty or so billion cells be dead in order to make a diagnosis of brain death? If not, which functions may remain? For example, in the most tragic "locked-in" syndrome, all means for communication except movement of the eyes and eyelids is lost irretrievably because of brainstem infarction. The patient can hear and see but can neither speak nor move. Some cannot swallow; others have difficulty with respiration. Such patients can be maintained alive for months; in many, their respiration persists, their brain waves may be nearly normal, they are conscious. The costs of maintaining such patients in the Intensive Care Unit and the emotional drain on the family are incalculable, while the eventual outcome is certain. Yet they are not dead and few physicians are willing actively to extinguish such lives. I believe the reason is that mind and consciousness persist.

A lesion but an inch away results in permanent coma without any chance for recovery of consciousness; yet such patients maintain their vital functions intact. Their EEGs are quite abnormal — not flat however. They may exist equally long in Intensive Care Units with the same eventual outcome, but here a neurologist might part company with his other medical colleagues and with the public in considering such patients to be dead because of their permanent loss of mind.

A lesion slightly higher may be associated with retention of consciousness without comprehension — so-called akinetic mutism. Such patients have their eyes open but are totally unresponsive. One particularly tragic example of this condition came to my attention when an out-of-state doctor wrote me, requesting suggestions for any new treatment he could try for his patient. The patient is a three-year-old boy who nearly drowned about six months previously and who has been comatose since then, exhibiting all the signs of akinetic mutism. Can conscious but mindless persons be considered dead? If so, where will we stop?

A patient paralyzed and speechless may live for years, a burden to his family, a drain on scarce facilities, useless, forgotten, and neglected. My department recently received a letter from a woman who is having to face this kind of bleak situation. Her husband had a stroke nine months ago and has been totally disabled since then. He was hospitalized twice, for 51 days initially and for over a month later. To pay the hospital bills, she has depleted her savings, and to care for him at home, she has had to quit her job. He is paralyzed on one side, cannot speak, and must be fed through a tube. The doctors say he will never recover.

Would it be better for these patients to die, and should a neurologist accelerate the process? A similar question could be asked of the senile and the severely retarded. Yet we are repelled by the idea, often not so much because it violates our moral values, but because we fear where such a policy might lead.

A recent report[32] indicates that patients who suffer cardiac arrest and subsequent coma have a poor chance of recovery without severe intellectual impairment. In an editorial about this problem, the *Lancet* states that survival of such patients is worse than death. "When coexistent causes (metabolic, postcardiosurgical) are absent, coma after cardiac arrest is a sign that further resuscitation attempts . . . may be misplaced."[33]

In the past, the physician's sole aim was to avert death and induce recovery, in many cases at great expense in manpower and resources of the family, the hospital, and sometimes the community in general. With the advent of the concept of brain death, however, a new dimension will be added. The neurologist will be called to the bedside not only to cure but to kill.

This abrupt departure from a tradition thousands of years old bring physicians and society face-to-face with an issue that has been smouldering some 20 years. What should be their attitude toward patients whose existence is maintained by using respiratory and, in some cases, cardiac and vasopressor support, when, after a reasonable length of time, no evidence of brain recovery is apparent? We have all seen or heard of instances when patients remain in coma for months to years requiring around-the-clock nursing care and expensive support systems, who occupy scarce hospital beds, and whose maintenance exhausts the families' emotions and finances. Wouldn't it be easier simply to certify such patients as dead?

Dr. John Skillman has stated that physicians must face certain problems posed by their unwillingness to discontinue life-supporting help in terminally ill patients.[34] They may be rightly concerned about their own patients, maintaining them in an Intensive Care Unit (ICU), but, in doing so, they exclude other patients from receiving this kind of care. As he says, "the very reason for intensive care is to provide the best chance for those whose illness is catastrophic but not necessarily lethal. . . . When it is clear that a patient has no chance for recovery, the continuation of intensive care becomes a mockery"[35] of the efforts of the medical staff. The choice of patients for admission and discharge to an ICU should be based on a consideration of which patients have the best chance of useful survival. Note the word 'useful.' Brain death seeks to resolve the dilemma posed by keeping cardiorespiratory vegetables "alive" in ICUs. The insertion of 'useful' adds another dimension to the problem, a judgmental one that has caused an enormous soul searching on the part of physicians charged with responsibility for selecting patients to occupy scarce ICU beds. Generally speaking, stroke victims cannot compete for such beds.

Although neurologists always attempt to spare the family and society excessive emotional trauma and expense, they have traditionally made their decisions for the benefit of their patients. Now for the first time, they must decide for the benefit of others, for society and, in the case of cardiac transplantation, for another patient to whom they have no responsibility whatsoever. Here they may stand isolated from other physicians whose patients' survival may be dependent upon the neurologist certifying his patient is dead.

Furthermore, under reasonably similar circumstances, equal pressure may be exerted to declare a patient alive, as in the case of patients whose condition results from secondary complications of surgical procedures and in whom surgical success is equated with survival, even in a comatose state.

No longer is death an all-or-none affair with a dividing line agreed upon by all of society including its physicians. The neurologist and neurosurgeon are asked to make a judgment about which there can be argument and about which not all physicians and not all of society would agree. We will be asked to divide patients into three categories: those whose bodies and brains are alive, those whose bodies are alive but whose brains are dead, and those in which both are dead. This seems reasonable at first glance, but the consequences of this initial step in the redefinition of death are vast and frightening. Aside from the legal implications[36] of certifying persons dead when their body function and metabolism can be maintained, one must face immediately the awful realization that the brain does not die as a unit, that the most recently evolved portions are the first to die and the last to recover in instances of brain anoxia, so that all gradations and degrees of brain death are possible. Granted that even though today we accept as the criterion for brain death only total loss of function at all levels, it will be a reasonably simple matter to adjust this definition to suit changing needs in the future. After all, killing people is murder only when the law defines it as such. If physicians were given legal sanction, death could be made speedier for many patients, and, in many cases, this would be a blessing for all concerned. However, it could be but a matter of time before the enactment of the next step, that is, certifying patients who are permanently comatose or who are permanently mindless as also legally dead.

Physicians are already questioning the thesis that a person can be declared dead if he exhibits irreversible coma or brain death in addition to a lack of spontaneous respiration and a flat EEG, whereas a person is alive even though irreversible neocortical destruction has been confirmed if he still breathes spontaneously. These definitions exist in spite of the fact that the mind of the latter patient is dead and cannot ever recover. One report questions this arbitrary distinction between "alive" and "dead" as attaching "cardinal importance to the function of respiration and none to those higher functions of the nervous system that demarcate man from the lower primates."[37] Could not such patients be declared legally dead with the stroke of a pen? What of the aments who populate our state mental institutions? Such patients are also a drain on the family and on the sources of society. They too have a hopeless prognosis. As a matter of fact, the donor of the world's second cardiac transplant performed on December 6, 1967, was an anencephalic infant. All that is necessary is for the legal definition of death to be changed to include those who have non-development of or irreparable loss of higher cortical functions. At the present time these segments of our neurologic population are out of sight because they are out of mind. Loss of such functions can be assessed. This argument smacks of euthanasia, but so does the certification of a patient as dead when his heart still beats. Euthanasia is murder only so long as society deems it to be and killing becomes murder only when society makes it a crime.

Different Philosophies at the Bedside

One very practical but unanticipated aspect of the brain death concept is the unique vantage point of academic neurologists for watching the interplay of the various philosophies that people bring to the practice of medicine. We have idealists, usually medical students who want to keep the patient "alive" at all costs. We have more experienced physicians, who embrace with enthusiasm the now eight-year-old concept of brain death. But most enlightening of all, we have house officers from various parts of the world and, in my department, Americans, Europeans, and Asians, Catholics, Jews, Protestants, Hindus, and Moslems and, I suspect, a scattering of atheists. By academic tradition, decisions relating to patient care are discussed openly and opinions concerning proper methods of treatment are arrived at by persuasion, citation of literature, and only as a last resort by professorial pronouncement. However, with the newer concepts of death, personal attitudes, not technical knowledge, are the mode, and, as a consequence, each one's point of view has equal weight. The well-advised professor of neurology is not dogmatic, so that many a patient who might otherwise die is kept alive because of one therapeutic enthusiast.

One case illustrating this problem involved a man of 82 who developed hemiplegia and aphasia due to a stroke. His family and the referring physician both suggested that the man had lived a full life and that no heroic measures should be undertaken to keep him alive unless full recovery was likely. The patient was admitted to the Intensive Care Unit where immediate measures for protection of the brain were instituted. By policy, I have insisted that all patients, no matter how gloomy the outlook, receive 72 hours of intensive therapy just to be certain that we are not overlooking a treatable problem or one in which an unexpected recovery might occur. In this instance, the patient showed no sign of recovery and after seven days developed pneumonia because of aspiration from his tube feedings. Immediately the house officers started antibiotics, intravenous fluids and positive pressure ventilation. I, as attending neurologist, suggested that the antibiotics should be stopped, but patients in Intensive Care Units receive intensive care. To move him out would suggest defeatism and insult the ethic and conscience of some physicians. Everybody agrees that cardiopulmonary resuscitation should not be undertaken in the event of cardiac arrest, but antibiotics are an everyday measure. Can one legitimately withhold this standard treatment? Untreated, pneumonia would be a quick and easy means for allowing the patient to die. In this case, the patient received antibiotics and after three months is semicomatose and abandoned by his family. Discussions with my friends from other countries where antibiotics are a rare resource indicate that antibiotics would be considered heroic treatment and would not be given in such an instance. What is an ordinary treatment in one location is extraordinary in another, in effect situational ethics applied to decisions relating to death.

Another actual case that caused a conflict among my staff members might be instructive. A 63-year-old man was admitted to the hospital and diagnosed as suffering from amyotrophic lateral sclerosis, a remorselessly progressive wasting of muscles that kills slowly and agonizingly by paralyzing swallowing and eventually respiration. During his hospital stay, his heart unexpectedly stopped and the nursing staff immediately instituted resuscitative measures, after which they called my house physician. He immediately contacted the family to determine their wishes regarding the choice between sudden death from cardiac arrest or slow death in about six months from suffocation. As this caused some delay in the doctor's reaching the hospital, the nursing staff was furious, believing that his first priority at all costs should have been to save the life of the patient. This illustrates the kinds of conflict that may arise among the members of a medical team. The nursing staff felt the patient should be saved at any cost; the attending doctor believed the family's wishes should be ascertained first.

CONCLUSION

Where will all of this lead? The outcome is uncertain but one thing seems clear. The public must be made aware of the pragmatic difficulties involved in deciding the issues of brain death and death with dignity when the fate of actual patients hinges on such decisions. Increasingly, physicians and particularly we neurologists will be faced with extraordinarily complex issues with which we have not been trained to cope and for which we have little stomach. The public must be willing and prepared to accept part of this burden.

Even the issue of "death with dignity" is controversial. Is dignified death possible today when modern medicine can prolong life artificially for months and even years beyond its natural end? Paul Ramsey believes the term is fallacious, that "there is nobility and dignity in caring for the dying, but not in dying itself" and calls death instead "the final indignity."[38] Others disagree,[39] believing one can still die with dignity. Clearly the physician must attempt to promote as much dignity as possible for dying patients in spite of undignified circumstances.

These issues will be debated for some time to come. In the meantime physicians must exercise great caution in classifying patients as hopelessly ill. For example, it is my belief that many of the "hopelessly" deteriorated patients in nursing homes are in fact not suffering from brain deterioration so much as social deprivation. With the new concept of brain death, accurate diagnoses for all patients are more imperative than ever before. We cannot afford to neglect those patients who are capable of rehabilitation even as we attempt to make death easier and quicker for the many others who are terminally ill.

The physician's primary responsibility is still to cure. Patients consult him for this purpose, not for diagnostic data that they can use to make their own decisions. If the physician tells the patient there is "no cure," the patient is disappointed and depressed but he can learn to accept it with time. Time is the crucial element in allowing patients to accept such situations. To tell the patient and his family that the prognosis is hopeless, however, can be devastating. Dealing with patients and families sympathetically will always be important. Even with obviously hopeless diagnoses, few patients ask to die, and those who desire to do so have ample means at their disposal with which to accomplish this goal. The physician may not aid anyone in this attempt as society has proclaimed it illegal. From my experience in dealing with such patients, I have found that they are often depressed and may be making a dramatic act in order to gain attention for solution of a problem. If the problem is solved, the desire for death disappears.

Physicians have indeed become too scientific, that is, too detached and objective. We use the scientific approach and abandon the art of caring for patients to nurses. What patients want is understanding and sympathy, and a good physician enthusiastically accepts this role as part of his responsibility.

The new brain death criteria can be an important step forward in medicine, one that can benefit patients, families, and society alike. Both professionals and laymen must be involved in deciding these issues so that a consensus can be reached that will be humane, moral, and ethical for all concerned.

NOTES

Acknowledgments — Mrs. Peggy Gratz, Editorial Assistant, Medical Library Bowman Gray School of Medicine was extremely helpful in the preparation of this manuscript.

1. Francis W. Peabody, "The Care of the Patient," *Journal of the American Medical Association* 88 (1927): 877.
2. Charles D. Aring, "Intimations of Mortality: An Appreciation of Death and Dying," *Annals of Internal Medicine* 69 (1968): 137-52; idem, "The Value of Life," *Man and Life: A Sesquicentennial Symposium* (Cincinnati: University of Cincinnati, 1969), pp. 1-4; Daniel Silverman, "Cerebral Death — The History of the Syndrome and Its Identification," *Annals of Internal Medicine* 74 (1971): 1003-05; and W. Russell Brain, *Mind, Perception, and Science* (Oxford: Blackwell Scientific Publications, 1951).
3 Henry K. Beecher, "Ethical Problems Created by the Hopelessly Unconscious Patient," *The New England Journal of Medicine* 278 (1968): 1425-30.
4. Ad Hoc Committee of the Harvard Medical School to Examine the Definition of Brain Death (Henry K. Beecher, Chairman), "A Definition of Irreversible Coma," *Journal of the American Medical Association* 205 (1968): 337-40.
5. *Black's Law Dictionary*, 4th ed., s.v. "death."
6. Ad Hoc Committee of the Harvard Medical School, "A Definition of Irreversible Coma," pp. 337-338.

7. Alexander M. Capron and Leon R. Kass, "A Statutory Definition of the Standards for Determining Human Death: An Appraisal and a Proposal," *University of Pennsylvania Law Review* 121 (1972): 90.

8. A. Christian Compton, "Telling the Time of Human Death by Statute: An Essential and Progressive Trend," *Washington and Lee Law Review* 31 (1974): 532.

9. *Kansas State Annals* §77-202 (Cum. Supp. 1973) and *Maryland Code Annals* art. 43, §54F (Cum. Supp. 1973).

10. Compton, "Telling the Time of Human Death," p. 536.

11. Capron and Kass, "A Statutory Definition of Death," p. 109.

12. *Ibid.* p. 109-110.

13. John J. McCutchen, "A Neurologist Looks at Death," *Journal of the American Medical Association* 204 (1968): 1197-98.

14. American Medical Association, "Report of the Judicial Council on Death" (1973).

15. Ad Hoc Committee of the Harvard Medical School, "A Definition of Irreversible Coma," p. 339.

16. Capron and Kass, "A Statutory Definition of Death," p. 100.

17. Euthanasia Educational Council, "A Living Will," (revised 1974.)

18. Lucy G. Morgan, "On Drinking the Hemlock," *Hastings Center Report* 1 (1971): 4-5.

19. Lawrence K. Altman, "A Fatally Ill Doctor's Reactions to Dying," *The New York Times*, July 22, 1974, p. 26.

20. Capron and Kass, "A Statutory Definition of Death," p. 91.

21. *Ibid.* p. 94.

22. John D. Arnold, Thomas F. Zimmerman, and Daniel C. Martin, "Public Attitudes and the Diagnosis of Death," *Journal of the American Medical Association* 206 (1968): 1949-54.

23. Ad Hoc Committee of the American Electroencephalographic Society on EEG Criteria for Determination of Cerebral Death (Daniel Silverman, Chairman, Michael G. Saunders, Robert S. Schwab, Richard L. Masland), "Cerebral Death and the Electroencephalogram," *Journal of the American Medical Association* 209 (1969): 1505-10.

24. J. B Green and A. Lauber, "Return of EEG Activity After Electrocerebral Silence: Two Case Reports," *Journal of Neurology, Neurosurgery and Psychiatry* 35 (1972): 103-07.

25. The first electroencephalographer, Hans Berger, was troubled by the ethical dilemmas of performing EEGs on the dying and had this to say:

    The ability of the brain to function is first extinguished in the youngest and last in the oldest parts of the brain. Till now I have always declined to follow the suggestions made to me from various sides subsequent to reports on my investigations, that I should study the gradual extinction of the E.E.G. in a dying person, for I hold such investigations to be inadmissable on moral grounds. However, years ago I already had observed the gradual extinction of the E.E.G. in the animal experiment and had found that the alpha-waves coalesce more and more, becoming longer and flatter, similar to what I have been able to observe in pathological cases. . . . The animal no longer reacts to any stimuli. The E.E.G. progressively approaches a straight line on which the very much slowed single oscillations are only recognizable as very feeble deflections. One may assume that in the dying human the E.E.G. behaves in the same way as is shown in the dying dog. There too, during the gradual extinction of life, the alpha-wave will probably become progressively slower and of smaller amplitude, until the galvanometer records only a straight line as an indication that the cerebrum has irrevocably ceased its activity.

Pierre Gloor, "Hans Berger on Electroencephalography," *American Journal of EEG Technology* 9 (1969): 76.

26. R. Bickford, "When Is Death? Computer Assessment of Brain Damage," Inaugural Lecture, University of California, San Diego, November 8, 1969.

27. M. Brock, A. Schurman, and J. Hadjidimos, "Cerebral Blood Flow and Cerebral Death," *Acta Neurochirurgica* 20 (1969): 195-209.

28. J. M. Goodman, F. S. Mishkin, and M. Dyken, "Determination of Brain Death by Isotope Angiography," *Journal of the American Medical Association* 209 (1969): 1869-72.

29. H. Arnold, P. Ansorg, P. Voigtsberger, and H. Eger, "The Determination of Brain Death and the Consequent Identification of the Time of Death by Means of Pulsatile Echoencephalography," *Acta Neurochirurgica* 27 (1972): 263-75.

30. Rick Edmonds, "Girl Is Alive Here After She Was Declared Dead," *Winston-Salem Journal*, July 27, 1974, p. 2.

31. James F. Toole, "Danger Ahead: Problems in Defining Life and Death," *North Carolina Medical Journal* 28 (1967): 464-66; idem, "The Neurologist and the Concept of Brain Death," *Perspectives in Biology and Medicine* 14 (1971): 599-607.

32. J. A. Bell and H. J. F. Hodgson, "Coma After Cardiac Arrest," *Brain* 97 (1974): 361-72.

33. "Coma After Cardiac Arrest," *Lancet* 2 (1974): 1302.

34. John J. Skillman, "Ethical Dilemmas in the Care of the Critically Ill," *Lancet* 2 (1974): 634-37.

35. *Ibid*, p. 636.

36. Because the moment of death becomes arguable, it raises the specter of a number of medicolegal complications.
    1. In inheritance cases when two persons suffer fatal trauma, the determination of precedence of fatality can be extremely important.
    2. Insurance policy complications can arise.
    3. The timing can be adjusted for the convenience (or at the expense) of one or more parties because neurologic consultation and special diagnostic aids are not always available.

37. J. B. Brierly, J. H. Adams, D. I. Graham, and J. A. Simpson, "Neocortical Death After Cardiac Arrest," *Lancet* 2 (1971): 565.

38. Paul Ramsey, "The Indignity of 'Death with Dignity,'" *Hastings Center Studies* 2 (1974): 48.

39. Leon R. Kass, "Averting One's Eyes or Facing the Music? On Dignity in Death," *Hastings Center Studies* 2 (1974): 67-80.

ROBERT P. HUDSON

Death, Dying, and
The Zealous Phase

Suddenly death never had it so good. Was it only five years ago
that one could lament that Americans employed massive denial
to avoid all truck with the subject? That they refused even to
consider the possibility of personal mortality, and consequently
managed it badly when the end finally came? That one reason
they invested $1200 per average funeral was to assuage their
guilt and fears?

Well, the Old Black Nemesis ain't what she used to be. Dying
is in, providing of course it is accomplished with dignity. What
was once tabooed is now widely discussed. It has arrived on
campus: this year more than 70 undergraduate courses will
explore dying and death,[1] a phenomenon featuring the creation
of instant academic expertise to a degree unmatched since the
professors discovered Black Studies in the late 1960's. Without
actually counting, it appears there will be more conferences on
dying this year than on human sexuality, and one must wonder
if that can be healthy. The literary magazines are forced to
review new books on death a covey at a time. There are at least
three periodicals devoted to the topic, *Omega*, the *Journal of
Thanatology*, and the *Journal of Life Threatening Behavior*.
There is a massive bibliography compiled by HEW and another
by the University of Minnesota, meaning, one supposes, that it is
only a matter of time until scholars in this area will have to begin
their endeavors with a MEDLARS search. And surely the
Euthanasia Educational Fund must be struggling to meet the
demand for Living Wills. If progress in the field depended on
exposure, then certainly we have turned a big corner. It is not too
early to begin worrying that the subject may soon (forgive me) be
talked to death.

Getting people more friendly with death was a necessary first step. As a matter of fact, in several important aspects we are well past the talking stage and into the action phase. The public is accepting the notion that death should be as dignified as its essential ignominy permits. They no longer insist that life be extended without regard to its quality. This is not to suggest that the war is won. Many physicians continue in the grand tradition, pushing the button for a "Code Blue" resuscitative effort with no more intellectual expenditure than Pavlov's dogs invested in salivating.

Although acceptance of the importance of personhood and the quality of life is by no means universal, it has progressed far enough to guarantee a continued spread without much further nagging from theologians and ethicians.[2] In truth, history will show that the public led the medical profession in the current trend toward more reasonable practices regarding dying patients, which is probably as it should have been. Just as the law properly follows social consensus, so too should medical practices, at least in such essentially social matters as who may end life and when.

History teaches a lesson at this point which may have something to say to the sudden popularity of death and dying. The lesson relates to what may be called the zealous phase of social or scientific discovery, 'zealous' here being used in its sense of excess. The adverse effects of new ideas come not when they are being propounded, but in unwise or premature application after the idea gains a foothold. The first phase, that of debate, generally is one of harmless abstractions. The second stage, acceptance and application, is one of deeds, and thereby more susceptible of abuse.

It has been relatively recently that mankind has come to see that adverse social consequences frequently follow scientific discovery. That phenomenon can be viewed as a variant of Newton's Second Law of Thermodynamics and, with quantitative apologies, reads: for every scientific action there is an equal and opposite social reaction. For one simplified example we can point to the connection between Fleming's discovery of penicillin in 1929 and the passage of the Medicare Law in 1965. Penicillin helped keep alive thousands of older persons whose susceptibility to expensive chronic illness pressured society into a new method of financing health care for the elderly.[3]

The process of social reaction to scientific discovery, at times inherently hurtful, is exaggerated by unwarranted or premature exploitation of new scientific developments. Scientists have been as guilty here as have consumers of science. Within one year after Rudolf Virchow demonstrated the power of pathology in understanding the development of disease, microscopic enthusiasts described the brain lesion specifically responsible for suicidal behavior.[4] Pasteur and Koch had no sooner proved the germ theory of disease causation, than others triumphantly announced the isolation of germs causing cancer, multiple sclerosis, and a number of diseases whose causes remain unknown still today.[5] Zealotry can flourish at times even if the initial "discovery" was totally erroneous. In 1903 the distinguished physicist. M. René Blondlot, claimed he had discovered a new ray, which he called N-ray in honor of Nancy, the city where he was working. His discovery was confirmed by others and the many physical properties of the amazing rays were determined, including the fact that they played a fundamental role in the biological as well as physical world. The list of contributors included some of the foremost scientists of the time: Jean Becquerel, Gilbert Ballet, André Broca, Zimmern, Bordier and others. What a pity that a short two years later the whole subject area was abandoned. In Rostand's words. "N-rays, N7-rays, and physiological radiations would never again grace the pages of scientific journals, in which they had cut so marvellous a figure."[6]

The same phenomenon marks major advances in dealing with those conditions which present ignorance leads us to describe as non-organic mental illness. Nineteenth century alienists, as psychiatrists were then called, took a giant step toward humane treatment when they led society to accept the idea that many alcoholics, kleptomaniacs and other victims of compulsive behavior were ill, not merely criminal. The zealots soon rode in however. One result was the concept of masturbatory insanity, a diagnosis that put many perfectly healthy young people in mental institutions, some for life.[7]

One could go on to no particular end. The purpose of this historical preface is not to bad-mouth science, but to show how zealous abuses can grow out of legitimate developments. The balance of this essay will explore several areas in which the field may be joined by well-meaning, but potentially counterproductive enthusiasts.

The first such area involves the specialists, i.e., the metaphysicians and health professionals working in death and dying. One danger here lies in the quest for semantic and conceptual precision in clinical situations characterized by biological imprecision. The concept of personhood, now in vogue, can serve as an example. No one seriously disputes the value of the current dialogue on personhood.[8] The human womb at times discharges a deformed creature that must be called human life because it is just that, a live product of a human zygote. The more extreme of these so offended our professional progenitors that they labelled them monsters. Even today they are so alien to the norm and totally devoid of potential that they evoke different semantic treatment. The purpose of holding that they lack personhood is to confront the biological fact of human life in a way that permits a different moral treatment. The monster is human, but not a person. Broadly applied, the notion of personhood would seem to be useful here.

But there are limits to the application of personhood that cannot be overcome. The term can never provide physicians or others with the precision necessary to set down workable guidelines governing every decision to abort a fetus or invoke euthanasia in the dying aged. The basic and unyielding reason for this is the incredible complexity, indeed uniqueness, of each dying situation. No two persons can die the same any more than they can live the same. Not only is each dying episode unique, it is also a process in time, so that the degree of personhood changes daily, whether the human being is developing or disintegrating. Thus a human trait that counts toward personhood one day can become a minus the next — sensitivity, for example, after the development of bone pain from metastatic carcinoma.

Draw up your choicest list of qualities conferring personhood and you have a house of cards. The final definition fails because the qualities involved are not points but ranges on a spectrum, ranges whose lower and upper limits themselves defy specific fixation. One such list (making no pretense at completeness) includes 1) self-awareness, 2) self-control, 3) memory, 4) a sense of futurity, of time, 5) a capacity for interpersonal relationship, 6) love, and 7) desire to live.[9] Applied to a healthy newborn baby, there is no convincing proof that 1, 4, 5, 6 or 7 are present; at the very least, we lack the means of demonstrating them. Never to my knowledge has memory (3) been verified before age one and it is rare that a person, without reinforcement throughout childhood, can recall events before age three. And most parents will agree that item 2 is irritatingly absent in the neonate.

Are we to conclude then that the newborn does not possess personhood? According to one version of the current wisdom, not at all. Personhood is there, but it is not yet demonstrable. The newborn has the *potential* for personhood and therein lies the critical distinction. Potential becomes the saving concept. In its 1973 abortion decision, the Supreme Court was driven to this word when it indulged itself that remarkable demonstration of logical legerdemain which had them modestly denying their ability to determine life's beginning, but unequivocally fixing the "potential for life" at the start of the third trimester.[10] Here is precisely the sort of nonsense that often devolves when we attempt to impose legal precision on biological processes. Legislators willing to rewrite their abortion laws in accordance with the wisdom of the Supreme Court will find no practical way to fix the "potential for life" (beginning of viability), because there is no biological point that fixes the beginning of the third trimester. The best the obstetricians can do in a given case is an estimate that varies plus or minus 2-3 weeks.[11] Even if medical science could fix precisely the beginning of the third trimester, it would be useless for the purpose at hand. It would be a calendar date, i.e., the number of days from conception, and in certain instances would bear no relation to fetal viability, because the various organ systems do not always develop at the same rate. The only certain way to determine viability is to remove the fetus intact by Cesarian section and make every attempt to sustain its life, a solution of dubious value in the abortion question.

The personhood concept exhibits the same deficiencies in a dying adult. Suppose we agree on the seven qualities listed above as minimal to a definition of personhood. Our agreement only begins the difficulties. Do we mean total or partial presence of a given quality? How do we quantify self-awareness? Does the total permanent absence of memory end personhood? If so, how long must it be absent to be permanent? In short, what combination of which qualities to what degree must be present to signify continuing personhood?

All that is being said here is that if one has in mind guidelines for abortion or euthanasia, personhood confers no more precision than did the older word, life. This is not to say the newer term is useless. On the contrary, its heuristic value is great and derives from the stimulus it gives to *attempts* at separating suffering or vegative life from the reasonaby pain-free, thinking, feeling form. The point is only that we must acknowledge that the matter cannot be resolved by physicians or metaphysicians apart from the sickbed. Personhood is a useful abstraction, but provides final resolution only in extreme situations precisely because it is an abstraction, and one that defies final definition even as that.

Whether personhood (or its potential) exists will be decided by a complex combination of medical and socio-economic considerations played off against the personal convictions of the dying person and his loved ones *as they face an imminent death*. The same combination of circumstances will never occur again and by extension, the same definition of personhood will never be repeated. All of this, of course, is old to those embroiled in the revival of situational and contextual ethics, but there appears to be a recurrent need to emphasize the unpredictable nature of biologic and medical variations that will always thwart those who seek a single metaphysical system to cover all clinical situations, while providing the Linus' blanket of absolute internal consistency.

There is a growing need for physicians to know in advance the circumstances under which a given patient would prefer that heroic therapy not be invoked. One such mechanism, the Living Will, has stimulated wide popular interest in recent months. With this document, the patient effectively attempts to define what he means by a dignified death. Copies are filed with his physician, his lawyer, and other appropriate persons. The intent is not to bind the physician legally, which probably would not stand the test of law, but to free him morally at a time when the family is under great duress and the patient may be unable to make his wishes known. On the surface, well and good, but contrasting two such Living Wills can again illuminate the pitfalls inherent in striving for precision in such matters.

In the version offered by the Euthanasia Educational Council the operative sentence reads, "If there is no reasonable expectation of my recovery from physical or mental disability, I, _____, request that I be allowed to die and not be kept alive by artificial means or heroic measures." The stipulations have the merit at least of brevity and a saving vagueness. "*Reasonable expectation?*" "Physical or mental *disability?*" "*Artificial* means?" "*Heroic* measures?" These terms involve what is referred to in athletic contests as judgment calls, the question, for instance, of whether a tennis ball touched the baseline. In tennis, we empower a single person with these arbitrary decisions. His judgment is final regardless of correctness. But tennis is not a dying matter, except perhaps for the few ultra-chauvinists who staked their manhood on Bobby Riggs over Billie Jean King. The judgment-calls specified in the Living Will are largely medical. They can be made only if the deciding individual understands fully all the medical aspects involved. In current practice this usually means the physician, whose duty then becomes that of educating the patient and abiding by his wishes. Whether patients want to or should invest such final trust in their physician, and indeed whether physicians want and merit the responsibility, is not the point here.

Look now at another Living Will, this offered by Marya Mannes in her book *Last Rights*. Five categories of disability are itemized, singly or together, as tantamount to a request for *active euthanasia*. Only the first three are quoted here, but the others are equally specific and thereby obfuscating.

1. Any disease or accident that would leave me unable to take care of my own bodily functions or deprive me of independent mobility.
2. Progressive deterioration of mind as evinced by total loss of memory, only partial consciousness, chronically irrational behavior, delirium, or any other evidence of advanced senility.
3. Any condition requiring the use — beyond two weeks — of mechanical equipment for breathing, heart action, feeding, dialysis, or brain function without a prognosis of full recovery of my vital organs.[12]

The attempt at precision in these provisions, laudable in its aim, would paralyze any physician into confused inaction. "Independent mobility?" A quadiplegic can operate a motorized wheelchair, while an individual with an optimally functioning artificial limb may require help to traverse certain terrain. Which, if either, is independently mobile? "Full recovery of my vital organs?" The loss of one lung may drastically reduce exercise tolerance, but allows a comfortable and long existence to those with sedentary occupations. Justice Douglas wore a cardiac pacemaker for years and continued to function to everyone's satisfaction, physiologically if not judicially. This is clearly "mechanical equipment," and the good Justice has zero chance for "full recovery." Would Ms. Mannes request death by committee action under these circumstances?

Which brings me somewhat reluctantly to active euthanasia. The August 1974 issue of *The Humanist* features a discussion of the subject by such stellar names as Joseph Fletcher and Daniel Maguire, names that promise the subject a measure of resurrection and serious discussion. The last previous push for legalized active euthanasia peaked in this country in the 1940s, but apparently the issue was not dead beyond the resuscitative powers of

today's philosophers and theologians. Active euthanasia will
have tremendous appeal for the zealots, and here metaphysicians are the least worry. Philosophers and theologians are an
independent strongwilled lot, and even when you get them
together for purposes of voting, a consensus is newsworthy and
unanimity a minor miracle. But legislators and social planners
are something else; by their nature, they are always meeting, and
for them compromise is a way of life. Active euthanasia is an
issue they can get their teeth into. As the number of old folks
increases and the cost of supporting their nonproductive existence increases, public pressure is bringing the question of voluntary active euthanasia back to the attention of lawmakers.

Fletcher reiterates what others have held, that there is no
moral difference between active and passive euthanasia, that the
end in each instance is the same, and that whether action or
inaction is the means, either is known to implement the desired
end.[13] But to agree there is no essential moral difference between
active and passive euthanasia does not rule out other important
distinctions. We need spend little time on the first and obvious
of these, namely that in every jurisdiction in the United States
active euthanasia is chargeable as murder. These are the laws
proponents of active euthanasia would strike down. It is well
documented that juries frequently acquit in so-called mercy
killings, even when the facts unquestionably demonstrate an
outright killing. In the famous acquittal at Liege, the mother
confessed from the witness stand that she gave her
thalidomide-deformed child a lethal dose of sedative. In a more
recent instance, a man dispatched his paralyzed brother with a
shotgun blast to the head in front of witnesses and was acquitted
on the wonderfully flexible grounds of temporary insanity. But
the fact that juries often acquit in these pathetic circumstances
should offer scant comfort to physicians who might, under present laws, entertain fleeting thoughts of active euthanasia.

Any system of voluntary euthanasia would demand stringent
legal controls. As usually conceived, this system involves some
sort of committee arrangement, presumably using guidelines,
which returns us again to the problem of semantic precision and
biological imprecision. In 1967 a furor erupted in London's

Neasden Hospital when a browsing patient discovered a directive posted for the staff indicating that the cards of patients over 65 with malignancies or chronic chest or kidney disease were to be marked "NTBR" — "not to be resuscitated" if they suffered a cardiac arrest.[14] Quite properly, the ensuing fuss finally focused not on any perceived callousness, nor on the decision itself not to resuscitate, but on drawing an arbitrary line at age 65. This is the sort of administrative insanity that must accompany the legalistic approach to the dying process.

The fact that an administrative setup will not work does not mean it will not be set up. On the contrary, joyous optimism in the face of repeated failure is a hallmark of social planning in recent years, witness crime, poverty and racial integration in the schools. If the enthusiasts are to be deterred in active euthanasia, positive steps must be taken. One beginning might be a determination of the actual need. How many persons must traverse a course of terrible suffering to find solace in death? No one knows, but in all likelihood the number is small. Certainly many are suffering needlessly at the moment. Since medicine's serious interest in the dying is a recent phenomenon, it is not surprising that the team approach to pain control is just now evolving. The principal problem is not the lack of means to ease the physical aspects of dying, but the lack of education and proper utilization. There is little taught on the subject in medical school. As incredible as it is on only cursory examination, too many physicians remain reluctant to addict their terminal cancer patients. Many Roman Catholics act as though they are unaware that in 1957 Pope Pius XII approved the use of drugs that shorten life if the primary intention is to alleviate suffering.

There are cultural problems as well. The national paranoia over drug use deprives physicians of heroin even though some believe it is the best agent around for managing pain without undue dulling of sensorium. The magnitude of the problem will be known only after there has been a thorough application of known pharmacological knowledge and existing surgical procedures. It makes no sense to create a cumbersome legal structure to control a situation that may be manageable largely by nothing more than a wiser application of medical methods at hand.

Another desideratum which will not be explored in detail here is a better press for suicide. Self-destruction has much to recommend it in situations of the sort generally cited to further the cause of active euthanasia. A serious drawback is that suicide requires consciousness and physical ability. It is possible, however, that many patients would not reach a helpless state if they were conditioned throughout life to look on suicide as an honorable alternative when a degrading death becomes certain and imminent.

There is another danger in reopening the vermian can of voluntary active euthanasia. At the moment there are mercifully few legal decisions governing what physicians may do under the heading of passive euthanasia. Any attempt to write specifics into laws governing active euthanasia would almost certainly spill over into the passive region. Presumably one must decide how far the physician acting alone can go in administering drugs that may unintentionally shorten life before deciding he must seek legal sanction for a drug that will end life intentionally. Many of the criticisms of past physician ineptitude are justifiable in this regard. But most physicians are susceptible to education which in these areas has been rudimentary at best. The alternative, legalized voluntary euthanasia, is of course almost totally untried.

We might end this necessarily contracted discussion of voluntary euthanasia by asking, "To what extent must we involve the physician at all?" Once a patient (or his family if he can not) elects active euthanasia, the responsible physician is not needed beyond his written opinion that the situation is indeed medically hopeless. In truth, there are reasons why he should not be involved in the final decision, just as we insist that the transplant surgeon not be allowed to fix the time of donor death. Certainly the patient's physician is not needed to carry out the execution. Any technician will do. No great skill is needed to hit a vein with a dose of morphine as thousands of addicts prove daily.

It can be argued that the profession's healing image will be needlessly damaged by participation in voluntary euthanasia beyond the initial opinion of hopelessness. For the same reason, some have urged physicians to get out of the wholesale abortion business; their medical skill simply is not essential. Any reasonably bright and dexterous high school graduate can be trained in the suction method of abortion in a month or two.[15] Beyond deciding there are no medical contraindications then, why involve physicians at all?

The hopelessness of a given case is a medical judgment. The decision to request active euthanasia is the responsibility of the patient or his family. The execution itself is a social function, of greater moment than, but quite analogous to, that of putting strays to death in an animal shelter. If the process is to be legalized, society should create a new specialty for this purpose, one unrelated to any of the existing healing professions. None of this speaks to passive euthanasia, which should remain the province of physicians because it requires medical skills and daily clinical judgments. A considerable part of healing derives from the patient's conviction that his welfare is the physician's overriding concern. Even though the patient's welfare is at issue in active euthanasia, there is a real and, as we have seen, unnecessary threat to the patient's trust if he knows that the same hand will guide the syringe of penicillin and that of euthanasia.

There is a creeping tendency for society to use medicine for purposes that do not put the patient's best interests first. If medical care must be used as political warfare, as we did in Vietnam,[16] the profession should dissociate itself publicly from such practices. The same holds for sterilizing mothers to decrease the welfare load, for psychosurgery aimed at rendering more socially acceptable behavior that is not a genuine threat to the individual or others. This is not to argue that medicine should not serve social ends, because of course it should. But these social ends are best served when they coincide with the individual patient's welfare. Professional perversion can result when the social goal becomes the principal or only determinant. We saw this perversion when ante-bellum Southern physicians assessed the intellectual attributes of Negroes in ways that justified slavery,[17] and again when German physicians furthered the Nazi notion of super-race and took part in the widespread "euthanasia" practices for individuals simply because they could not be properly nazified.[18] All of this is not an attempt to prejudice the case for voluntary euthanasia by tarring it with Nazi abuses of World War II. It is meant instead merely as an admonition that as active euthanasia becomes a matter for serious public discussion, the medical profession must guard against perhaps the most dangerous zealots of all, those who mean no harm.

Besides the search for non-existent precision, health professionals could enter the zealous phase in another way. It is a tempting step from the discovery that many dying persons derive psychological benefit from outside intervention to the conclusion that we must do something for all of them. There are at least three possibly erroneous assumptions in this logical leap. The first, and obvious error, is that all patients require assistance beyond what they or their loved ones can provide. The second is that in every instance where intervention is more or less clearly desirable, we know the proper form that help should take. The third is that when the first two are present, we have the right people in sufficient numbers to do a good job on the more than 5,000 persons who die daily in the United States.

No physician can practice long without being impressed by patients who die well on nothing more than their own inner strength. Not a few have prepared themselves psychologically years before the event. Others without extensive previous effort, find ample emotional sustenance in religious or philosophical wellsprings. Some are so self-sufficient that they devote their last weeks to comforting those close to them and helping them begin the grieving process. Knowing how to help a dying person requires a large measure of compassionate sensitivity, but recognizing those who need no professional help requires no less.

With her pioneering work on death and dying, Elizabeth Kübler-Ross rendered a great service.[19] Still the prophet's ultimate value depends on what others do with the gift as much as the nature of the gift itself. It will be remarkable if Dr. Ross' contribution is not perverted during the next few years. In truth, her conclusions lend themselves to a sort of cookbook approach to dying patients which may be positively harmful in the hands of those armed principally with ardor, the quality that for Ambrose Bierce characterized "love without knowledge."[20] Five stages of dying — a remedy for each. Repressed anger stage? Tear down all the get-well cards or throw a ballpoint pen at the next devil who walks through the door. Depression stage? Merely point out that it is normal to be depressed at the thought of dying — that if you were in their fix, you'd be depressed also and besides, take heart, the depressed phase comes just before acceptance, so all will soon be well. It does not matter that the prophetess herself has warned against such simplism; Freud did the same with psychoanalysis, and two generations of psychiatrists paid little attention.

We need not belabor the obvious fact that not all patients go lock-stepping through the five stages in indentifiable ways. More to the point — even if they did, we would not always know how to handle things in every patient apparently wanting our aid. A given stage can call for widely varying therapeutic approaches. In many instances, no one can know precisely what would best serve. This complexity was illustrated by a recent case, (I will call him Mr. Simon) a 56 year old Jewish machinist, who was dying of metastatic carcinoma of the lung. Despite little formal education,he was deeply schooled in classic literature and philosophy. (This knowledge was never in doubt after the first interview when he asked his visitor if he preferred Ciardi's *Dante* to that of the classical Cary.) His philosophical pursuits had estranged him from the religion of his childhood, and in fact the consultation had been requested precisely because he had made such a forceful case for rational suicide that no one knew quite how to deny his persistent requests for a handgun. A social worker had noted that he tended to intellectualize everything about his dying process. Though not stated, the implication here was that he could not reach the stage of acceptance until he abandoned his cerebral approach in favor of some sort of visceral revelation. This attitude is finely attuned to the current emphasis on emotion over intellect, and in many instances perhaps it would have been proper. In the present case there is good reason to doubt the desirability of such an attack. Every time a probe was made in that direction, Mr. Simon promptly returned to rational analysis. Several hours were spent asking what was the sense of it all, agreeing there might be none, seeing that there had to be or life became ridiculous, pursuing the alternatives if life was indeed ridiculous, deciding that one either resorted to faith or concluded that living itself was the only point of life and on and on. Early it came out that he was not quite certain that shooting was the best form of suicide. With such obvious ambivalence, this subject was ignored by the consultant and returned to only half-heartedly by Mr. Simon on two later occasions. If he wanted to talk about Socrates and the hemlock, should some therapist persist in saying, "Socrates is well and good, but how do *you* feel about *your* impending death?" Of course he was denying, but is that always bad? He had relied on rationality almost exclusively in attempting to understand life as it was presented to him. Was it proper to insist that he approach the even greater riddle of death in a totally different way?

This is not to say that everyone of stature advocates the emotional route as the only way to the acceptance stage of the dying process. It is only to say that a cookbook strategy leads naturally to recipes for managing each stage. The plea is only for that modicum of humility, the willingness to say, "we don't know yet," that would have spared medicine so many baneful excesses in the past. The systematic assistance of dying patients is an infant art. We must repeatedly ask ourselves, "Where is it written?" When we do raise the art to something of a science, almost certainly we will find that the infinite variability of human beings dictates that the cookbook here has no more validity than it does in prescribing digitalis to a patient in heart failure.

It is not the zealotry alone that worries, but its association with ignorance under the guise of instant expertise. This deception does not refer to the honest quacks who quickly infest any area of rapid expansion in medicine. The quacks at least have the merit of knowing they don't know. This may not control their activity, but it gives them a certain cunning about boundaries they may not cross without doing hurt — to themselves of course, which is their principal concern. The object of concern of the well-meaning instant thanatologist is the dying patient, and therein is the rub. One simply cannot read a few books and become proficient in managing the psychology of dying. Bedside training is necessary here just as it is in all clinical medicine. During the Zealous Phase there are no certified specialists and of course no standards. The publicizing of the void in terminal psychological care will attract numbers of practitioners limited only by access to patients in a remunerative setting. The potential for damage here is at least as great as it is when any untrained person sets up shop to help others with the emotional problems of living.

What has just been said may sound like preface to a call for limiting counselling of dying patients to present card-carrying physicians and ministers. No such thing. Any would-be counsellor must have a knowledge of pain management, but he need not be authorized to write a prescription for morphine. He must understand the shattering psychological effect of bone pain, but he need not be able to pick out bony metastases on the X-ray.

On the contrary, rather than retaining the counselling of dying patients within traditional disciplines, this would be a good time to branch out. The sheer numbers involved guarantee that traditionally trained workers will not be enough. It is time to acknowledge that personal traits and wide experience count more than formal training in dealing with many human problems. There is no doubt but that any number of barbers, bartenders, and housemothers would do a better job with dying patients than many physicians and ministers. There is also a chance here to experiment with the probability that dying patients can help each other. Many fatal diagnoses now carry a prognosis of 5-10 years, Hodgkin's disease for example. These individuals might not only help others, but as we learned with Alcoholics Anonymous, help themselves in the process. The success of the AA idea has spread to many similar endeavors. The movement should have been noticed by medical schools, but the practical impact has been negligible. How many medical faculties include a former alcoholic, or a cured junkie, or a successful graduate of Weight Watchers? Unless he also has traditional credentials, practically none. Would-be counsellors of the dying, even those well-trained, can expect the same initial cold shoulder from medical educators. They will be welcomed only when they can present meaningful certification and when existing disciplines realize that the newcomers present no serious threat to pocketbook or prestige. In the interim, the zealous phase, a certain amount of anarchical confusion is bound to occur. In any new field the first practitioners are by definition self-ordained. Their diploma is indistinguishable from that of any diploma mill simply because there are no accepted certifying agencies.

Another hazard derives from ordinary and understandable ignorance. Lacking medical knowledge, it is easy for a patient or family to give up before the situation is truly hopeless. Indeed, instances of this have already happened. This does not refer to the well-known and not infrequent situation wherein the family has ignoble reasons for wanting Granny in the grave. Rather, the reference is to zealots whose motivation is altogether compassionate. They talked it over with Granny on several occasions and everyone agreed that when her time appeared, there would be no medical heroics. At some point an apparently catastrophic event occurs, and the relatives promptly toss in the towel.

As a case in point, not long ago a physician received a long distance call from an elderly patient's wife. She requested medical blessing for her decision to do nothing for her husband who had just lapsed into coma following an earlier stroke that had left him slightly impaired but satisfied with life. The physician knew them as an intelligent couple who had made a considered decision that if the situation became hopeless, one partner would allow the other to die with dignity. He told his caller he was in complete philosophical accord, but that it was medically unsound to make such a decision by telephone. Reluctantly, the wife transported her husband to the hospital where he was found to have a chronic subdural hematoma. A neurosurgeon removed the blood clot and by all measurements the patient was returned to his previous level of health.

It might be argued that this example constructs a straw man, that no physician would ever pronounce medical hopelessness over the phone. Such sanguinity unfortunately is not supported by the facts. Physicians are no more immune to social pressures in their professional practice than ministers or lawyers. It is estimated that antibiotics are properly prescribed only one time in ten.[21] In the other nine are many instances of giving the antibiotic simply because the patient insists on having it. A good deal of morbidity results from this practice and even some mortality, but on it goes. Pressed about it, physicians frequently respond that if they don't give the penicillin, mama will take her child to a doctor who will. This defense has that certain charm that infects much ingenuous logic, but it has a pecuniary ring as well.

The point is that medical practice, while ideally patient-centered, is often influenced by unrelated social forces. It is not unlikely that if society becomes, shall we say, overly enthusiastic in the premature abandonment of older citizens, medical practices will accommodate in subtle ways just as they are now changing to meet the perceived social need for more dignity in the dying process and a move away from the use of technology simply because it is there. The unthinking physician, in the popular demand for a dignified dying process, will have to guard against contributing to premature deaths. We will have to remind ourselves, and the public, that death comes soon enough — no need to send out a posse.

The issues of death and dying have always fascinated theologians, philosophers and poets, but largely as abstractions. Since practical considerations were few in the past, the law has been involved only peripherally and in ways that offer little help in the complex and unprecedented ethical problems that characterize the scene today. Because the issues had little visible social impact, no existing discipline claimed them for their own. This essay has contended that the current burgeoning of interest in death and dying will result in a period of relative anarchy. Until the field clarifies itself and lines of responsibility can be drawn, it is vulnerable to overzealousness on the part of the public and its institutions, of which the healing profession itself is one.

NOTES

1. "Thanatology 1," *Time*, January 8, 1973. According to the Euthanasia Education Fund, the figure for 1975 is 112.

2. For a summary of attitudes toward death in 30,000 non-representative subjects see E.S. Shneidman, "You and Death," *Psychology Today*, June 1971, p. 43 ff. In a recent survey of 933 randomly selected physicians *Medical Opinion* reported 79% believed the patient had a "right to have a say about his own death." Reported in *Psychology Today*, September 1974, p. 29.

3. I have elaborated this theme in greater detail in "Action and Reaction in Medical Research," *Annals of Internal Medicine* 67 (1967): 660-67.

4. F.A.H. La Rue, *Du Suicide* (Thése pour le doctorate en medicine, Universite-Laval de Quebec) (Quebec: St. Michel et Darveau, 1859), p. 20.

5. The process actually began in earnest some forty years before final proof of the germ theory. See W. W. Ford, *Bacteriology* in the series produced by *Clio Medica* (New York: Hafner Publishing Company, 1964), p. 57.

6. J. Rostand, *Error and Deception in Science* (New York: Basic Books, Inc., 1960), p. 27.

7. This story is told in fine fashion by E.H. Hare, "Masturbatory Insansity: The History of an Idea," *Journal of Mental Science* 108 (1962): 2-25.

8. One of the best recent exchanges on the personhood concept appears in *Perkins Journal* 27 (Fall 1973). Particularly worthwhile are the articles on the beginnings of personhood by H.J. Taubenfeld (Legal), H.T. Engelhardt, Jr. (Philosophical), and A.C. Outler (Theological).

9. The first six of these were taken from J. Fletcher, "The 'Right' to Live and the 'Right' to Die," *The Humanist* 34 (1974): 15. In context Fletcher is questioning rather than denoting these as qualities necessary for personhood.

10. The companion cases of Roe v. Wade, 410 *U.S.* 113, and Doe v. Bolton, 410 *U.S.* 179.

11. P. Casaer and Y. Akiyama, "The Estimation of the Postmenstrual Age: A Comprehensive Review," *Developmental Medicine and Child Neurology* 12 (1970): 697.

12. M. Mannes, *Last Rights* (New York: William Morrow & Company, Inc., 1974), pp. 134-135.

13. J. Fletcher. See footnote 9.

14. "Resuscitation Edict Stirs a Storm," *Medical World News*, October 20, 1967, p. 54.

15. Or at least so I am told by a professor of obstetrics and gynecology at my parent institution.

16. E. Langer, "The Court-Martial of Captain Levy: Medical Ethics v. Military Law," *Science* 156 (1967): 1346-50.

17. As one example see A. Deutsch, "The First U.S. Census of the Insane (1840) and Its Use as Pro-slavery Propaganda," *Bulletin of the History of Medicine* 15 (1944): 469-82.

18. L. Alexander, "Medical Science Under Dictatorship," *New England Journal of Medicine* 241 (1949): 39-47. For insight into the subtle progression by which the Nazis gained control of German physicians see H. Bloch, "The Berlin Correspondence in the JAMA During the Hitler Regime," *Bulletin of the History of Medicine* 47 (1973): 297-305.

19. E. Kübler-Ross, *On Death and Dying* (New York: The Macmillan Company, 1970).

20. A. Bierce, *The Enlarged Devil's Dictionary*, ed. E.J. Hopkins (Garden City, New York: Doubleday & Company, Inc., 1967), p. 16.

21. H. Beaty and R. Petersdorf, "Iatrogenic Factors in Infectious Disease," *Annals of Internal Medicine* 65 (1966): 641-56. For evidence that recognizing a problem may do nothing to remedy it, see H.E. Simmons and P.D. Stolley, "This is Medical Progress? Trends and Consequences of Antibiotic Use in the United States," *Journal of the American Medical Association* 227 (1974): 1023-28.

DALLAS M. HIGH

Quality of Life and Care of The Dying Person

In this essay I shall attempt to discuss an important but difficult notion — quality of life of the dying person. It is important because it is sometimes hinted at in discussions of care of the dying, is attached to discussions of health care delivery, and is becoming an underlying aim of the practices of such institutions of care for the terminally ill as St. Christopher's Hospice (Sydenham, England). Moreover, it is becoming widely known that dying patients usually do not fear death so much as they fear pain, isolation, physical deterioration, and that dying is a brutal assault on one's general well-being. Dying is feared because it usually means that life's quality will be lowered to a point of becoming intolerable. It is a difficult notion since as a society we have found it increasingly difficult to talk about quality questions. "Quantity questions are much easier to decide," we say. Moreover, it is difficult because we live in an emergent society which has implicitly embraced an ethic of quantity of life (and so has embraced life prolongation techniques). The current imperative is "One ought to live long," and it is often embraced at the expense of or in disjunction from "One ought to live excellently." Many may even find it odd to join together "dying" and "quality of life" questions. Therefore, it may be useful at the outset to discuss some manifestations of the cultural sensibility which gives the issue at hand its peculiar context.

Life as The Highest Good?

There is currently a remarkable obsession with talking of death and dying in Western culture. We are daily told that "death has become a taboo"; we are told of cultural and individual fears and denials of death; and in some lecture circuits the subject of death

85

is now outdrawing the perennial crowd pleasers — politics and sex. It may not be unfair to say that the current obsession, in American culture at least, is an attempt at exoneration from Arnold Toynbee's famous charge that "death is un-American and an affront to every citizen's right to life, liberty and the pursuit of happiness." There is evidence to believe that interest in the subject has already produced a consensus that death ought to be accepted. Sometimes it is remarked that death is as much a part of life as birth and sex. But, this is a move which takes for granted that the questions of what it means to say "I was born" and "I will die" (the timeful dimensions of my own life and mortality) are settled as simple biological processes. The move then readily turns one to questions of technological man-agement of a dying patient and even to a sensibility to "over-come death" by an effort to prolong "life" indefinitely.

Long before the current death and dying obsession, Hannah Arendt in her significant work, *The Human Condition*, recognized the philosophical and cultural features of modernity prompting such moves. Our difficulty is that we can easily confuse the delineations of life and death since we presuppose a world in constant change and espouse the possibilities of man-agement of human existence as a laboring animal.

> . . . the turning point in the intellectual history of the modern age came when the image of organic life development — where the evolution of a lower being, for instance the ape, can cause the appearance of a higher being, for instance man — appeared in the place of the image of the watchmaker who must be superior to all watches whose cause he is.
>
> Much more is implied in this change than the mere denial of the lifeless rigidity of a mechanistic world view. It is as though in the latent seventeenth-century conflict between the two possible methods to be derived from the Galilean discovery, the method of the experiment and of making on one hand and the method of introspection on the other, the latter was to achieve a somewhat belated victory. For the only tangible object introspection yields, if it is to yield more than an entirely empty consciousness of itself, is indeed the biological process. And since this biological life, accessible in self-observation, is at the same time a metabolic process between man and nature, it is as though introspection no longer needs to get lost in the ramifications of a consciousness without reality, but has found within man — not in his mind but

in his bodily processes — enough outside matter to connect him again with the outer world.[1]

What is remarkable in our time is not simply that we have seen scientific endeavors combat disease, relieve suffering, prolong life and delay death, but that these efforts are directed toward cutting the tie of life from our earthly nature and to making life artificial or controllable. Says Arendt,

> It is the same desire to escape from imprisonment to the earth that is manifest in the attempt to create life in the test tube, in the desire to mix "frozen germ plasm from people of demonstrated ability under the microscope to produce superior human beings" and "to alter [their] size, shape and function"; and the wish to escape the human condition, I suspect, also underlies the hope to extend man's life-span far beyond the hundred-year limit.[2]

To be told that "death is simply a part of life" and to attempt to gain acceptance of death on that premise may well be an attempt in management. In other words, such acceptance may be seen as an attempt to escape the human condition with an assertion of the ongoing process of life, whatever its definition, as the highest good. It is at this juncture we need to look carefully and critically at what Elizabeth Kübler-Ross and others have embraced as a "stage of acceptance." It may be more closely akin to a "state of bankruptcy."[3] It is in this sense that efforts which finally glorify and beautify death can be seen as efforts to assert life as the highest good so that it becomes increasingly difficult to discern whether life is worth living or not. That is to say, life becomes a temporal but qualitatively neutral notion. Says Arendt, "No matter how articulate and how conscious the thinkers of modernity were in their attacks on tradition, the priority of life over everything else had acquired for them the status of a 'self-evident truth'. . . ."[4]

The current problem is not simply about travesties caused by the so-called life-prolongation techniques of an aggressive and zealous medical urge to "preserve life at all costs," but it is as much, if not more, a question concerning what modernity has tacitly embraced or tended to include in what is meant by life and death.[5] If a patient is urged to accept death, does this mean he should accept life as well? In what way? Or is it asking individual patients to embrace "life" and "death" as a single natural force? Such a force is appropriately described as "the force of the life process itself, to which all men and all human activities [are] equally submitted ('the thought process itself is a natural process' [Marx]) and whose only aim, if it [has] an aim at all, [is] survival of the animal species man."[6] None of the higher capacities of man (claimed by tradition and antiquity) nor any of the struggles and defiances of man are any longer necessary to individual life in its connection with species and the world. If this is so, there is emerging on our cultural scene a strange, but unacknowledged, alliance between those who espouse accomplishment of a stage of acceptance of death and those who urge "mercy killing," i.e., death is a beautiful part of life.[7] The claims that death is a part of life, or that death is a disease which somehow needs to be treated or even cured or passively accepted as a chronic condition are, at best, instructive only of the symptoms of a cultural sensibility.

So far I have neither made an argument for nor against a reverence for or sanctity of life, and I have not intended to imply such comments. Rather, my claim is that the primary problem is that of recognizing and acknowledging the sense and meaning of death and the quality of life of sufficient dimensions to remain conceptually distinct from death. Questions of denial and acceptance of death are only secondary questions, if questions at all. Leon Kass appears to be correct in claiming that the question of dignity or indignity of death is a misplaced question and should not arise even though the question of dignity is closely tied to how one lives or is allowed to live, including how a dying patient lives, "though merely to live is not yet to live excellently or with dignity. . . ."[8]

Failure to take note of the current cultural sensibility has, I think, contributed to a rash of pseudo-questions, often taken as genuine moral dilemmas, such as, "To treat or not to treat a patient"; "Turn off the machine or not turn off the machine"; or false alternatives as (1) life prolongation; (2) active intervention to end life; (3) passive management, i.e., shortening the dying process.[9] I shall now turn to these matters in an effort to discuss them as concretely as possible, but I shall claim that such questions become significantly moral questions only as we concern ourselves with the quality of life and not with mere life and its possible duration. What possibly could be the intrinsic worth or value of life as a form of calendar counting of years?[7] If one drops the time-oriented conception of life and death as the primary concern, then it is less a question of how long one will live and more a question of how easy or difficult living will become for a dying person.

To Prolong Life?

Robert H. Williams, M.D., in his prologue to the book *To Live and to Die: When, Why, and How*, offers a curious claim which, if followed, produces chaos in the care of the dying. He says, "There are times when the merits of dying outweigh those of living. Sometimes we have gone to unwise extremes in unduly delaying death. There are times to promote living and times to promote dying."[10] This is an odd claim even if well intentioned. Williams' claim confuses dying and death.[11] If one correctly distinguishes dying and death, then it is almost self-evidential that one should never "promote dying" or claim that dying, as such, has any merits about it, especially if the latter is always distinguished from living of a sufficiently high quality. For example, one should never deliberately stimulate cancerous growth in order to produce a terminal illness. No one rationally desires to be in a state of dying or have a terminal illness, just as most people do not enjoy being ill. Persons, however, may want to die. That is, people sometimes do express a desire to be dead rather than to live, but not to be in a state of dying. The expression of a desire to be dead, rather than to live, is essentially an expression concerning the relative insufficient quality of one's existence (life). Moreover, it is most often not a fear of death which troubles the fatally ill as the prospect of a lowered quality of life during the course of dying, e.g., assault of disease, pain, isolation, dependency, physical disfigurement, etc. Although we cannot morally claim dying as a desired state, we can talk morally about the quality of life (and care) of the dying. I shall return to this subsequently.

My point now, however, is that without careful attention to appropriate distinctions, oversimplistic jargon clouds the issues, as if the only alternative question was to prolong life or not to prolong life. Even though, for example, St. Christopher's Hospice in Sydenham, England is viewed by me, after a personal research visit, as a place I would want to be cared for if I should be dying of cancer, I do not desire nor can I rationally desire to check into the men's ward of the Hospice for a two-week period of dying, as if to take a two-week vacation comparable to an excursion to the seashore at Brighton, England or Myrtle Beach, U.S.A. The situation is far more sober than any glibness which attempts to glorify dying and death or make places for the dying appear sentimental, warm, and motherly. Such processes of thinking have given rise to the extreme positions in care situations: (1) Aggressive and heroic procedures and efforts to prolong life at all costs where anything short of that is held to be a failure. (2) Omit or withdraw all treatment of the dying and/or urge the legal acceptance of killing the dying patient.

With the above extremes as a background, some moralists and physicians have attempted to delineate courses of action in moderation. A good example of that position is an essay by Vincent J. Collins, M.D., in which he subscribes to a guideline of "passive management," that is, to draw a limit to life prolongation and shorten the dying process. To quote, "When one permits death by not continuing therapy, the harm that is done is done by nature acting. This is passive management based on reason and judgment — and shortening the act of dying."[12]

In order to maintain such a position there must be a defense that it is morally correct to "shorten the dying process." Presumably, Collins wishes to distinguish "shortening" the dying process from both "ending" it and "lengthening" it. His claim is based on "permitting nature to take its course" as decided by the effectiveness of therapy and the distinction between ordinary and extraordinary means. The latter distinction, given by Pope Pius XII, is well known and highly debated. I shall not rehearse those debates here. It suffices to note simply that defining "ordinary" and "extraordinary" according to the circumstances is at best difficult and variable. Moreover, even if this is done in practice, it can only take us so far. For Collins, extraordinary means are those which sustain life artificially in order to buy time for "natural restorative processes to operate." This definition will hardly evoke widespread agreement, since a number of means are, indeed, proper without any hope of natural restorative processes, nor will it take us very far in support of passive management of the dying as either morally correct or as a proper medical procedure. Even with these difficulties, the distinction about means has received an honored place in medical practice. In 1974 the House of Delegates of the American Medical Association, after making a disclaimer of mercy killing, continued its statement with the following:

> "The cessation of the employment of extraordinary means to prolong life of the body when there is irrefutable evidence that biological death is imminent is the decision of the patient and/or his immediate family. The advice and judgment of the physician should be freely available to the patient and/or his immediate family."[13]

Richard A. McCormick appropriately remarks of the statement that it fails in essential ways to address the shifted state of the questions. The questions are not always "Is this means too hazardous, expensive, or painful?" or "Will this means offer no reasonable hope of healthy benefit and only protract dying?" Basically the questions have shifted, argues McCormick, to the following kind: " 'Granted that we can easily save the life, what kind of life are we saving?' This is a quality-of-life judgment."[14] Of equal difficulty are the references to the well-worn but confusing notions of "life of the body" and "biological death." As recent discussions indicate, the latter notion may be a meaningless locution in reference to persons.

A Right Time To Die?

An interesting proposal has recently come from some of the people who have been directly involved in care of the terminally ill. It is that there is "a right time to die." Although nowhere to my knowledge is this view fully explicated, it trades on some form of claim that death is natural and urges careful and comprehensive medical diagnosis which is respective of a patient's age, health, maturity, and life style in determining the right time. Moreover, this claim seeks to rebut procedures and actions which artificially hasten death or shorten the dying process as well as those which protract dying. To quote Richard Lamerton,

> "It is proposed that there is a right time to die; that this time may come before a man has breathed the very last breath of which his body is capable; and that an experienced physician can recognize, or learn to recognize, that this right time to die has come. Please understand that what is proposed is to refrain from prolonging life beyond the right time, NOT to hasten the termination of life in any way."[15]

Put forward in just this way Lamerton's claim could mislead in at least one feature, namely, that a right time to die is when one's life is no longer productive, or the right time to die is before winter sets in. (A farmer friend during my childhood days would always comment on an April or May death in the neighborhood, "I can't understand why a person would die in spring after already making it through a hard winter.")

Lamerton's claim is made mainly in reference to the physician's or care professional's responsibility and judgment — but such a judgment should not be set apart from a sensitive understanding of the patient's individual needs and sense of self, including one's own (my own, to put it in first person) life story, style, purpose and aspirations. I may well have some sense of a well-timed death, but what is most difficult is for others to tell me (or know) what that is. We do know that elderly people will often make the point that they are "ready to die," but the care professional's problem is to know how to respond to that. The ethical problems arise when one attempts to determine that a certain medical practice has become "meddlesome medicine" with regard to a timing of death and what kind of response a care professional should make to the dying person's sense of life story and end of that story. Lamerton says, "When a patient is seen to be preparing for death, this is something we [physicians] should respect."[16] In addition to the variety of ways one can accord respect, it is also the case that one may (or I may) prematurely "prepare for death." Such situations could arise in at least two ways: mistaken understanding of my own diagnosis and prognosis, or factors of depression, anxiety and pain resulting from my inability to cope with my illness and/or deficient care. Lamerton cites two cases in support of his claim of a right time to die, one of which he concludes by saying ". . . she died at the right time of pneumonia, which we did not try to cure."[17]

It is not difficult to present counter cases which propound the ethical difficulties with the "right time" claim, especially when judgments are made in highly interdeterminate situations. However, the basic difficulty of the notion is that it does not provide an ethical guide in care of the dying. That is to say, it does not provide a foundation upon which to say what ought to be done before the right time is known or what ought to be done well in advance of the right time. Most likely it is the case that an individual's quality of life, sense of well-being, and personal achievement are the factors which actually provide the basis for a biographical account of a well-timed death. Consequently, good care for the dying person may be the aid to a sense of a death well-timed, not that a right time to die determines the mode of care.

Personal Well-being While Dying

All too often the terminally ill are referred to as "hopeless cases" which have to be "managed" under the condition of "life decline." I want to claim that such references and practice-orientations are ethically misguided. But let me first focus on what we can call the "life decline" model of dying. My claim is that a goal of proper care and a morally high quality of life of the dying should not stand on an easy acceptance of such a model. Robert S. Morison appropriately describes what regularly guides our outlook upon or model of the dying person in the following:

> "The life of the dying patient becomes steadily less complicated and rich, and, as a result, less worth living or preserving. The pain and suffering involved in maintaining what is left are inexorably mounting, while the benefits enjoyed by the patient himself, or that he can in any way confer on those around him, are just as inexorably declining."[18]

While Morison is correct to claim that these are "the unhappy facts of the matter" in most situations, it surely is not an ethical claim that this is how matters ought to be (prescriptively) or that these are unalterable facts of the matter. My concern here is that too much attention has been paid to taking these "unhappy facts of the matter" as unalterable givens and then responding to them on the basis of arguments about euthanasia, limits of life prolongation, and attempts to distinguish "ordinary and extraordinary means" and "omissions and commissions." Too little attention has been given medically and ethically to altering the "unhappy facts."

It is my judgment that the "unhappy facts" can be altered, at least to a significant degree, in many if not most cases, and that the "decline" model does not have to preside over an ethic of care of the dying any more than we should confuse aging with dying or an irreversible illness with insufficient well-being. One can recognize that a person is terminally ill (chiefly a diagnosis by a physician), but that does not negate either a viable quality of life until death or conditions of care to "live well" to the end. The "life decline" model regularly equates life with biological or physiological processes which may be deteriorating. But this equation needs to be challenged since a viable quality of life always involves more than these processes and, as a result, necessitates comprehensive care for the entire person. A dying person's lament that "everyone is hurrying about awfully concerned about my liver, my blood, the IV's, etc., but no one seems to be concerned about me" is germane.

Comprehensive care for dying persons is almost entirely a new phenomenon. Not only is it well known that most of medical education is directed to acute care and little attention is given to training in care of chronic or terminal illnesses, but there has been a relatively significant shift since the turn of the century in the causes of death (terminal illnesses). There has been dramatic shift from communicable diseases to chronic degenerative diseases (diseases of the heart, cancer and other malignant tumors, cerebrovascular diseases). This shift means that more often than not, the dying process (not to be confused with aging) comes later in a life span and that for all there is an increased possibility (and accompanying fear) of a long and painful dying process. Moreover, it is clear that more and more people are "doing their dying" in hospitals or in other institutions and are consequently living their last days removed from the familiar and the usually friendly environs of home. Relatives are more frequently unwilling or unable to take on any role of responsibility in coping with the terminal illness of a loved one in part because the public is increasingly impressed with "life saving" techniques and the patient management abilities of hospitals and institutions.

Any discussion of comprehensive care for the dying person should not attempt to provide a rigidly formulated set of principles, for at least two reasons. First, it is well recognized, or at least widely assumed among the best of care professionals, that the individual identity of the patient is important. Second, there are always individual patient conditions and needs as well as individual purpose and life style of the patient up to the end. By the very nature of what constitutes the human condition of dying, including the condition of defining dying by the imminency of death, comprehensive care which is fully relevant and appropriate to the needs and style of the patient should be a primary concern.

If I have an inoperable cerebral tumor, for example, the care concern should not simply or always be to administer dexamethazone to reduce the fluid around the tumor and, hence, the pressure. My personal sense of well-being while dying will include (and as proper care for me, should include) relief from other distressing symptoms, pain, and fear of pain. This care might well include relief of the discomforts (often overlooked) of constipation and relief of other secondary symptoms. Moreover, I would have need of and would want an environment where my "dying needs" can be met without fear of being a burden. It should be an environment where my own integrity and responsibilities as a person (a comprehensive entity) have the fullest opportunity of expression and acknowledgment. I should be provided with the opportunity and freedom to voice my fears, my depressions, and be helped to cope with myself and my illness in the company of friends, family, and the care-team. This picture presents us with more than a care of primary symptoms or, medically, a biophysical dysfunction. It means simply that any ethic of care in which I, as a dying patient, am permitted to live with quality to the very end will give full and relevant attention to matters which extend beyond and are not exhaustible by physiochemical, physiological, or neurological needs and symptoms, whether or not one invokes the ambiguous, and perhaps bogus, distinctions between ordinary and extraordinary means (and care) and acts of omission and commission. (My argument implies, but it is not argued here, that the development of an ethic of care for the dying on discussions of the above alleged distinctions is misguided.)[19]

It is not only that I (and each human being) can lay claim to my need, want, and desire of *self* importance and a sense of meaningful relationships, but because I (and each of us) can lay claim to what it means to exist and, while facing death (dying), what it means to cease to exist.[20] If I am a comprehensive entity, not only does this mean that the so-called "brain death" is problematic as a concept of death, but what my needs for care are in the face of death are not simply so-called "vital" functions. If the meaning and significance of living, even while dying, can be assessed only by appeal to higher order operational principles, then discernment of proper care of the dying human being demands an exercise of ever more personal faculties. As a result, at least two features arise from this situation concerning the dying, and both are value-laden and evoke moral responses. First, the physician and entire care-team have responsibilities for decisions and judgments which attend to indeterminate and unspecifiable features — concern for quality of a human life as well as its length. Second, the important and, indeed, "vital" needs of the dying may often be those which extend beyond the mere physiological functioning, i.e. the needs of a living comprehensive entity, a personal subject. That is why the common literature offers criticism of reductive care of a patient since a patient is then being treated as a thing or object and not as a subject.

In a dying person, for example, the physiological functioning may be failing and unresponsive to any efforts aimed at alleviating the primary condition or disease. (Cancer patients often "watch" and sense the deterioration of their bodies.) Yet, it is clear that this same situation does not also mean that the comprehensive entity (the human subject) is unresponsive. It does not ever mean that "Nothing more can be done for a patient." The concept of care in the practice of meeting the needs of the dying is inextricably related to the concept of person; after all, persons, not organs (as entities in and of themselves), are finally the care concern. Of course, if one searches to define descriptively and exhaustively the characteristics of "personhood" and then attempts to insert those characteristics into clinical practice under the guise that more precision is being offered, one is bound to fail. However, the failure is not with the concept of person but with the lack of recognition and acknowledgment of the inexhaustible range of unspecifiableness and indeterminateness which makes care for human beings a moral and creative response, not the management of a "natural" and cyclical process. If a person is more than a collection of organs, tissues, behavior and dispositions to behavior, etc., then the primary objective in an ethic of care for the dying is the well-being of the comprehensive entity, the individual or personal subject. If the concept of person is not reducible to parts and sum of parts of an organism, but is of a higher order (an organism as a whole), then care for a dying person must proceed on those terms, that is, in terms of the person.

The case is, of course, appropriately parallel to the value-laden structure of defining death. Just as a reductionistic concept of death will not do, so too a reductionistic ethic of care for the dying will not do. Hans Jonas has argued persuasively that it is to "the organism as a whole" that we may properly apply the term death and not to some or all parts of an organism. This entails, as he further argues, that

> "my identity is the identity of the whole organism, even if the higher functions of personhood are seated in the brain. How else could a man love a woman and not merely her brains? How else could we lose ourselves in the aspect of a face? Be touched by the delicacy of a frame? It's this person's, and no one else's." [21]

To give intrinsic elusiveness its due is not being elusive relevant to making death decisions and decisions concerning care for the dying. Both are value-laden decisions and attend to an indeterminate range of moral responsibilities concerning the meaning of death and the quality of life. Neither can, therefore, be replaced by the mechanics of a value-free routine or a so-called morally-neutral care system.

To care for a person and to be cared for entails a proper and primary valuing of a person as a self-identical being. The level of well-being, and the patient's sense of it, should be the primary concern in the case of the terminally ill. The physician, the entire care-team, the family, the friends bear responsibility for aiding and providing conditions for the continued or even increased sense of well-being of a dying person. Concurrently, a dying person should not be relieved of all responsibilities; rather, one should be supported to assume responsibilities and manage oneself and personal affairs — all as appropriate and relevant to the condition of the patient. A general principle of "don't trouble him with that now, he's dying" only lessens the sense of integrity and well-being. It is clear that a dying person can always have a sense of purpose and self-esteem even though the mode of dying will be as individual as the person himself.

I recall visiting a patient at St. Christopher's Hospice, a patient who had been admitted some few weeks earlier with a diagnosis of terminal cancer and a prognosis of life expectancy of twelve weeks. When admitted she was suffering from unbearable pain, was extremely anxious about her impending death,[22] was constipated, and had a number of facial skin "sores," as she put it, which distressed her greatly. "I am sure that no one wanted to look at me," she said. "Even I couldn't bear to look in a mirror." The proper and relevant concern here was to treat, relieve and control the symptoms, not the primary disease. The primary concern was, and should be, for the individual person and that person's well-being and sense of well-being. When I last talked to the patient, her face was clear, she could apply her make-up daily, she was free of pain, etc. She said, "I feel good. I feel alive. I am happy even though I know my disease is spreading. Don't you think I look good?" She died a week later — "looking good." This vignette is, of course, illustrative. However, it is not an uncommon possibility, but is instead, in individual ways, a repeatable one, given proper and relevant care (treatment) of patients. Says Cicely Saunders, "We have to concern ourselves with the quality of life as well as with its length . . . These are not 'untreated' patients but rather those who have received the treatment relevant to their condition and so often to their wishes." [23]

Ethical Suggestions

As one concerned with the moral problems relevant to the quality of life of the dying, it is neither my province nor competence to recommend medical protocols and the details concerning patient care. However, I can argue, on ethical grounds, that more can be and should be done than is currently practiced. Therefore, having argued for a ground upon which to construct an ethic of care for the dying which is relevant to the quality of life of the dying person, I shall offer a principle and some guidelines. As ethical reflections, what I offer are statements of what "ought" to be, not what is practiced currently in all cases. I should also note that my reflections here are influenced by an effort to extrapolate some underpinnings of the practices of the hospices, such as St. Christopher's.

While it may be true that a terminally ill person has reached a point when no known cure is possible (or better, when it is known that there is a low probability of successful treatment of the primary illness), it is never true that "nothing more can be done." As a normative principle, we can then say, while one cannot always treat a primary, terminal illness or circumstance successfully, one can and should always *care* for the person until the very end of that person's life. Care is not an empty or sentimental notion. Rather, in the words of Cicely Saunders, it "should be full relief [of pain and symptoms] combined with a capacity to enjoy friends and food and all of the activity that is possible." Furthermore, care should often be delineated from hope of life prolongation, which is too often premised on "the only hope is to try a new, experimental therapy." A hope of living my remaining days (whatever they are) in a meaningful way is a positive alternative to choosing a difficult therapy at high risk. There is a need for skillful diagnosis and moral judgment when in an individual case aggressive medicine will likely become meddlesome medicine. It is never true that the only ethical alternative for a patient is either to give consent to an experimental therapy (a last "hope") or choose death. I can always assert the ethical propriety of wanting to die peacefully or live out my remaining days meaningfully, even in full recognition of a serious or dangerous illness. The patient, relatives, and care-team professionals should recognize that hope and meaning are not always predicated on the length of life. Quantity-oriented procedures should not occur at the depreciation of quality-oriented care. Under proper care, the terminal days can be and most frequently are the most meaningful for a patient and the relatives. Moreover, a physician's or care-team's attendance to the dying person can be a privilege, not merely a job. This does not minimize the responsibilities and dilemmas faced by physicians and the need for prudential judgments, but it does emphasize the importance of facing squarely the questions of quality and meaningfulness in human life. One patient at St. Christopher's Hospice, after wrestling with and working through her own recognition and acceptance of her imminent death, and achieving, most importantly, a reconciliation with her husband, remarked, "The last few days have been the most meaningful of my life."

Without offering some practical suggestions or guidelines, any principle can readily become platitudinous or an inutile ideal. For the remainder of this essay, let me sketch some open-ended guidelines aimed at the optimum of interface in delineating the ethical concerns of the quality of life of the terminally ill. It is hoped that these guidelines may serve, if nothing more, as a basis for further professional and public discussion of an increasingly important issue.

1. The dying person should be accorded respect, dignity, and a sense of self-integrity with purpose and fulfillment to the end of life.

2. All symptoms should be treated and controlled, as long as possible and as long as such treatment provides comfort to the patient. For the well-being of a dying person, it is important to realize that an appropriate therapy (and often, the only proper therapy) is symptomatic treatment. Often the care-team will

have to use all its skills possible to bring comfort to a patient, treating each symptom as it arises.

3. The dying person should live out the remaining days or weeks with minimal or no pain and remain, as fully as possible, normally alert. Pain is the symptom we usually fear most, but there is already considerable evidence that in most cases pain can be controlled, anticipated and prevented by proper drug regimens.[24] However, this ethical suggestion does underscore the need for additional research into the development of drug regimens and education of the public on their use. For example while diamorphine has been used successfully in Great Britain to prevent pain in patients with terminal malignancies, it remains an illegal and little understood drug in America, primarily due to widespread improper uses and "street" connotations of the drug. It should also be mentioned that it is often contended by moralists that there is a moral dilemma over administration of increased dosages of analgesics and narcotics in the relief or prevention of pain in the dying. That is, it is often asserted that the use of such drugs in increased dosages, in order to free the patient of pain, will hasten death. There may not be a moral dilemma here at all. R.G. Twycross, Pharmacological Research Fellow at St. Christopher's Hospice, informs me (verbally) that there appears to be evidence in his studies that just the opposite is the case. If drugs are administered properly, and especially administered as a pain preventative regimen (not P.R.N.), there is no evidence that death is hastened; rather, life may be lengthened in a way which is essentially pain free. To adopt the principle "Save the morphine (or diamorphine) until things really get bad" is a bogus principle both as it affects the dying person and his or her relatives.

4. The dying person should have the opportunity to clarify relationships, to continue friendships, and develop new friendships. The dying person should know the truth about himself even though oftentimes much skill will have to be employed to assist the patient to know and accept the truth. Honesty should be practiced. Attending persons (the care-team and relatives) should not engage in evasions or deceptions. This can only add

to a sense of loneliness, frustration, and a sense of abandonment. Although the depth of understanding will vary greatly among different people, attending persons should listen carefully and sensitively.

5. The dying person, when possible, should share with relatives in planning intelligently for changes which death will impose on the survivors. Attending persons should be available for such assistance and share concern for the relatives, both during the process of dying and after death.

6. The dying person should be accorded a familiar environment, one with familiar things and familiar faces, or be accorded surroundings as nearly homelike as possible. The appropriateness of this guide is already well discussed in a variety of places and needs no further discussion except to remind ourselves that it still remains badly followed.

7. The dying patient should be accorded the right to make care requests, to refuse treatment, to be consulted about his or her care, and to voice (and be seriously listened to) how he or she feels regarding the current and changing state of well-being. That is to say, the patient has the right (and it should be upheld) to be active in the decisions concerning himself or herself as long as possible. Attending persons should not be overprotective of the patient or create a sense of unreality. To be *cared for* may be helpful and comforting; to be *taken care of* may be demeaning. And, of course, it goes without saying that neglect is never a proper guide.

8. Attending persons (care-team and relatives in their decisions) should never cause harm and lessen the well-being of the dying person by the initiation or continuance of useless or irrelevant therapies. The Hippocratic Ethic itself of "doing no harm" can be extended to doing all things essential and relevant to the needs and the solution of the patient's problems. For example, just because it is widely known that antibiotics can successfully treat pneumonia in most cases, it is not sufficient grounds either medically or ethically to initiate such treatment in all dying patients who develop pneumonia. It is not a question (a psuedo-question) of "to treat or not to treat," but a question of relevant and appropriate treatment which needs careful

consideration in each case. Medically, pneumonia in the terminally ill may be fatal in spite of antibiotics, and, hence, irrelevant; morally, antibiotics may be inappropriate since the injections alone, for example, may cause needless discomfort.

> "There are times when the treatment for a haemorrhage is not a blood transfusion with its attendant alarms but instead an injection and someone who stays there. There are infusions which should never have been put up, feelings of thirst can be relieved by the right use of narcotics. It is far better to have a cup of tea given slowly on your last afternoon than to have drips and tubes in all directions." [25]

It is clear that the recommendations I have made in the foregoing underscore the need for a reorientation of values in many, if not most, instances of care for dying persons. Of importance, too, are the questions of resources, public policy, and economic priorities, but I have left those aside in order to sort out the ethical dimensions. Moreover, what I have said in this essay is not intended to cover all instances of dying persons. However, I will stand on the claim that these recommendations can be extended to the vast majority of dying persons. The widely discussed claim for euthanasia (mercy killing), for example, may in final analysis be a misplaced issue and may be a question genuinely relevant only in a few instances. The wide-spread concern should be the medical and moral priorities concerning the quality of life in care for the dying; only then, perhaps, can we gain a better perspective on other issues concerning the dying person.

NOTES

1. Hannah Arendt, *The Human Condition* (Chicago: The University of Chicago Press, 1958), p. 312.
2. *Ibid.*, p. 2.
3. See Ronald Koenig, "Dying vs. Well-Being," *Omega* 4 (1973): 184.
4. Arendt, *The Human Condition*, p. 319.
5. See Dallas M. High, "Death: Its Conceptual Elusiveness," *Soundings*, (1972): 438-458.
6. Arendt, *The Human Condition*, p. 321.

7. See Paul Ramsey, "The Indignity of 'Death with Dignity'," *The Hastings Center Studies* 2 (1974): 47-62.

8. Leon Kass, "On Dignity in Death," *The Hastings Center Studies* 2 (1974): 73.

9. Cf. Vincent J. Collins, "Limits of Medical Responsibility in Prolonging Life," *Journal of the American Medical Association* 206 (1968): 390.

10. Robert H. Williams, in *To Live and to Die: When, Why, and How* (New York: Springer-Verlag, 1973), p. 2.

11. See Leon Kass, "Death as an Event: A Commentary on Robert Morison," *Science* 173 (1971): 698-702, and High, "Death: Its Conceptual Elusiveness."

12. Collins, "Limits of Medical Responsibility," p. 390.

13. Quoted in Richard A. McCormick, "To Save or Let Die," *The Journal of the American Medical Association* 229 (1974): 174.

14. *Ibid.*

15. Richard Lamerton, *Care of the Dying* (London: Priory Press, 1973), p. 75.

16. *Ibid.*, p. 76.

17. *Ibid.*, p. 77.

18. Robert S. Morison, "Death: Process or Event?" *Science* 173 (1971): 696.

19. In my judgment, it is unfortunate that Paul Ramsey, in his *The Patient as Person* (New Haven: Yale University Press, 1973), attempted to develop an ethic of (only) caring for the dying (Chapter 3) by employing these distinctions. In order to make his case for a "patient centered" ethic, he has had to force equivocations and inconsistencies in the use of the distinctions.

20. In my "Death: Its Conceptual Elusiveness" I have argued that death is not a reductive concept and, as such, is value-laden. To recognize and to certify death is a taxonomy involving judgment of tacit dimensions which are never exhaustible by criteria. I still stand by that argument, but I would now modify my claim concerning the need for legislative statutes.

21. Hans Jonas, *Philosophical Essays* (Englewood Cliffs, N.J.: Prentice-Hall, Inc. 1974), p. 139. This is taken from his essay entitled "Against the Stream: Comments on the Definition and Redefinition of Death."

22. Most often pain and anxiety can only be artificially separated since the degree of pain and meaningfulness or meaninglessness of pain for a dying person is the way a whole person meets events of his life.

23. Cicely Saunders, "The Care of the Dying Patient and His Family," reprinted from *Contact Supplement* No. 38, p. 6.

24. See the following on the use of narcotics in preventing pain in the dying: R. G. Twycross, "Principles and Practice of the Relief of Pain in Terminal Cancer," *From the Postgraduate Centres*, July, 1972; "Clinical Experience with Diamorphine in Advanced Malignant Disease," *International Journal of Clinical Pharmacology, Therapy and Toxicology* 93 (1974): 184-198; Lamerton, *Care of the Dying*, Chapter 9; C. M. Saunders, "Treatment of Intractable Pain in Terminal Cancer," *Proceedings of Royal Society of Medicine* 56 (1963): 191.

25. Saunders, "The Care of the Dying Patient and His Family," p. 6.

JOHN LADD

Positive and Negative Euthanasia

The question I shall discuss in this paper is whether or not there is any ethically significant difference between negative and positive euthanasia, that is, between 'letting a hopelessly incurable patient die' and 'killing' him. The issue involves such questions as whether or not there is any difference ethically between turning off a machine supporting a patient's life and not turning it on in the first place; between doing something positive to hasten a patient's death and simply letting him die, etc., etc.

It is a well-known fact that many practicing physicians lean heavily on the distinction in question. Polls of physicians indicate that a large proportion of them approve in principle and are willing to practice negative euthanasia, whereas only a small proportion approve or are willing to practice positive euthanasia. Many laymen also hold the distinction to be a helpful and valid one.

There are doubtlessly legal considerations operating here, for in American law at present positive euthanasia is clearly illegal, whereas the legal status of negative euthanasia is more' doubtful.[1] Therefore, an American doctor faced with a concrete decision as to what to do is taking grave risks if he overtly practices positive euthanasia; and, if there is a moral obligation to obey the law, he may have moral reasons for not practicing it even though in principle he approves. For our purposes, however, it is necessary to disregard the legal side of the question; being illegal does not automatically entail that an act is immoral. As we all know, the law is often backward and no more than a reflection of bigotry and vested interest.[2] In any case, ethical considerations are logically prior to legal ones and must therefore be discussed independently of the latter. Much of the confusion in medical ethics is due to mixing up ethical with legal

105

questions. (The prevailing tendency to convert moral into legal questions reflects the general atmosphere of uncertainty in this area and grows out of the need to find some sort of authoritative guide as a substitute for independent thinking. The frequent resort to theology may be explained in the same way.)

At the very outset, we should consider the possibility that the distinction between positive and negative euthanasia is only psychological, that is, that the widespread acceptance of the distinction is rooted only in the subjective feelings of doctors and that as such it is to be explained by their distinctive personality, training or social environment.[3] If this argument is valid, then we can understand why it is so difficult to converse reasonably or philosophically about the distinction itself. Nevertheless, despite possible emotional blocks, it is most important for us to examine the distinction more carefully.

There are two extreme positions regarding the distinction between negative and positive euthanasia, "letting die" and "killing." Following Casey, I shall call them absolutist and consequentialist.[4] The absolutist position, which is advocated by most Roman Catholic theologians, holds that there is a significant difference between doing something evil intentionally and letting it happen as a 'by-product' so to speak. Killing an innocent person is always wrong, but allowing him to die may not be — under certain circumstances. (Like God who wills only good, but permits evil; man must will only what is good but may permit evil.)[5] The analysis offered of the distinction involves some questionable scholastic distinctions between different kinds of 'voluntary object,' 'intention,' etc.[6]

Intuitively (or psychologically!), it should be conceded, people often feel that there is a significant difference between making something happen and just letting it happen; for example, there seems to be an important moral difference between pushing a person into the river to drown and simply failing to jump in and rescue him if he accidentally falls in, i.e. letting him die.[7] But examples like this are tricky, for, without knowing anything more about the case, we probably instinctively take it for granted that there is a difference in motivation between the two cases: the man who pushes his victim into the water would have some kind of malicious motive, e.g. hatred, whereas the bystander who refuses to act might be motivated by indolence, fear or indifference. The trouble with carrying examples of this kind over into the medical sphere is that, as regards euthanasia, we hope to proceed with the assumption that there is good will on both sides. At least, in order to avoid extraneous considerations, we ought to assume that personal motivation, e.g., for killing or letting die, is not one of the issues.

Still, the intuitive approach to the problem is hazardous, simply because it is impossible to isolate an act per se in our imagination and consider it as such; some kind of background for the act is always part of the 'perception' of it. To use the Gestalt terms, every figure has a ground. By changing the ground it is easy, therefore, to change the 'perception' of the act. That is one reason why the relevance of the "euthanasia" activities of Nazi doctors is highly questionable; the motives of the Nazis cannot be compared with those of a doctor caring for his suffering patient. The motives are different, hence the cases are incomparable.[8]

The second position, that of the consequentialist, maintains that only the consequences of an act are relevant for determining the nature of the act and its ethical significance. Thus, if the consequences of two alternative acts are the same, to all intents and purposes the acts may be regarded as equivalent; if ostensibly similar acts (e.g., bodily movements) have different consequences, the actions are different. If ceasing to treat an incurable patient has the same consequence as killing him, namely, his death, then pro *tanto* the actions are the same. (There may, of course, be other significant differences, e.g. in suffering, in cost, or in saving someone else's life.) The virgins who threw themselves out of the window in order to avoid being raped, nonetheless killed themselves even though that was not their direct intention. For the consequentialist, the end-result is the only thing that counts.

Again, this position has some intuitive appeal. The parent, who hears that his child drowned while a bystander did nothing to save him, will justifiably condemn him as much as he would a person pushing the child in. From the victim's point of view, the

scholastic distinction may seem academic, if not cruel and in-
sensitive. Accounts of persons beseeching their doctors to put
an end to their misery are as persuasive and moving as any of
those accounts of feelings given on the other side.

It is or at least should be clear that we will not get very far if we
rely on "gut feelings" or "intuitions" for an answer to our
question. Yet, with a few notable exceptions, that is generally all
that we find in the literature on euthanasia and on the distinction between killing and letting die. Persons seem to feel that in
this area their feelings or intuitions have a special authority that
they don't have in other areas. But, inasmuch as the issues
involved here are basically ethical issues, the resort to *ipse dixits*
is entirely invalid, for we cannot resolve ethical questions by
appeals to "gut feelings," "intuitions," "self-evident truths,"
"dictates of conscience," or "God's word," etc. In order to ascer-
tain the legitimacy of such "evidences," we must already have
some sort of prior ethical standards.

Although the intuitive method, i.e., the appeal to self-
evidence, may be valid in perceptual or other kinds of knowledge, it is highly dubious in ethics. This is so for many reasons.
Appeals to "gut feelings" or "intuitions" simply confuse the
issue, particularly if the issue is precisely what the gut feelings
or intuitions are about! The obvious reason why simply "seeing
it to be so" (or "feeling it to be so") is not evidential in ethics is
that in ethical matters people "see" things differently, especially when the "seers" come from different cultures or from
different social classes. The analogy with perception is fallacious, for in perception there are standardized ways of accounting for error and for divergent opinions, for example, tests for
color blindness, defective hearing, etc. There are no such tests in
ethics. The analogy with vision has been refuted so frequently
and so thoroughly that it is hardly worthwhile to dwell on it any
longer. It should only be noted that the insistence on intuitions
(or self-evidence) as the foundation of absolute truth in ethics
simply invites all the usual arguments of relativism.[9] On the
other hand, if the appeal to intuitions or gut feelings involves no
claim to universality or objectivity, then it is hard to see how it
can have any bearing on the present debate: "this is what I

think" and "that is what you think" — so we reach an impasse or a *flatus vocis*.

The effect of basing one's position on "intuition" or "gut feeling" is to withdraw from the debate. It is a way of giving up or, if one wishes, of refusing to carry on the dialogue on an equal basis: "I have the intuition, you do not, therefore there is something wrong with you!" "I can see, but you are blind." Thus, there are ethical objections to the use of the intuitive approach as well as meta-ethical ones, for it indicates an attitude of superiority, a claim to privileged status, in ethical debate, a stance that is inconsistent with the categorical imperative. For, as Kant himself writes: there is a "duty to respect man even in the logical use of his reason: not to censure someone's errors under the name of absurdity, inept judgment, and the like, but rather to suppose that in such an inept judgment there must be something true," etc.[10] Thus, the appeal to intuition or gut feelings to settle an ethical controversy represents not only a breakdown in the argument but also a morally objectionable attitude towards those with whom one disagrees.

There are further meta-ethical objections to the intuitive method (and the use of gut feelings) in ethics. I can only briefly outline one of them here. It is concerned with the concept of moral neutrality, and, in particular, with how one goes about proving the moral neutrality of an act, activity, or state of affairs.[11] The logic of arguments of this type is as follows: in order to prove the moral neutrality of, e.g., an act, all that is required is to show that there is no reason for holding that act to be either right or wrong, that is, to show that the act in question has no right-making or wrong-making characteristics. Consider, for example, the proposition that playing tennis is morally wrong. How would one go about refuting such a proposition? One would obviously begin by asking: what makes it wrong? and, if no one can answer that question, the presumption would be that it is not wrong, and if it is also not right (i.e. obligatory), then it is morally neutral.

Gut feelings and intuitions are not the kind of thing that can *make* an act (activity, state of affairs) right or wrong. Hence, as such, they cannot serve as reasons of the kind required in an argument about moral neutrality. Hence, if there is nothing more that can be added, i.e., no further reason, why an act is right or wrong, then the presumption must be that the act in question is morally neutral.[12] For logical reasons, therefore, neither "intuitions" nor "gut feelings" are sufficient to establish the rightness or wrongness of an act; and, indeed, the implied denial that there are any other reasons leads to the paradoxical conclusion that the act in question is morally neutral.[13]

The upshot of this is that ethics operates under what I shall call the Onus Probandi Principle, the principle that the burden of proof rests on anyone who claims that an act, activity or state of affairs is morally right or wrong, good or evil, to show why it is to be considered so. In the absence of such proof, the presumption is that the act, activity or state of affairs is (in itself) morally neutral. An *ipse dixit* is not enough! Take, for example, the question of whether death is an evil or not. Anyone who asserts it to be (an intrinsic) evil assumes the burden of proof to explain *what makes it evil*. Sometimes, of course, it is easy to do this; but the categorical assertion that death is (other things being equal) always evil in itself may be no more than a piece of obdurate dogmatism or theological propaganda (or both!).[14]

Anyone who finds difficulty in accepting the Onus Probandi Principle, as outlined here, should think of how it operates in the law; for in legal proceedings, a claim without a proof is nothing more than a nullity. You cannot get by in the law by basing your claim on "gut feelings" or "intuitions" any more than you can in ethics. (I do not wish to suggest, however, that there are no important differences between legal and ethical arguments. There are, of course, many, the principal one being that there are no authorities in ethics.)

For the three reasons just given, any answer to our original question concerning the distinction between positive and negative euthanasia, insofar as it involves ethical issues, cannot be based on appeals to "gut feelings" or "intuitions," for "gut feelings" and "intuitions" provide no answer at all; anyone who uses them in an argument is guilty of an *ignoratio elenchi*. The Onus Probandi Principle requires us to give specific arguments, backed up by analysis and proofs.

With that in mind, let us begin by examining the concept of 'letting happen,' as it occurs in the phrase: 'letting the patient die.' First, it should be observed that 'letting X happen' is sometimes culpable, sometimes commendable, and sometimes neutral. Thus, in certain situations, the failure to act may constitute a form of negligence, even criminal negligence, as in the failure to take proper precautions with dangerous objects. Even in the case of death, someone who withholds something necessary, e.g., food or medicine, may be held criminally liable for a person's death.[15] To say that the doctor "let his patient die" is therefore not *ipso facto* a way of absolving him of culpability.

The question naturally arises: when and under what circumstances is "letting X (e.g. an evil) happen" culpable and when and under what circumstances is it commendable (or neutral)? We might begin by noting why people *do* let things happen (culpably). It is often easier to let something happen rather than intervene, e.g. out of laziness, cowardice or simply the desire to avoid committing oneself. Here one thinks of the Kitty Genovese tragedy, where numbers of people watched her being killed, *let* her be killed, without doing anything. The 'washing hands' motif is endemic in our society; whenever we can, we try to 'wash our hands' of responsibilities and commitments, especially if we are connected with formal organizations of one sort or another.[16] Perhaps this abdication of responsibility is the moral evil of our times, witness Nazism, Mai Lai, and Watergate; "I do my job and mind my own business, and I don't ask questions" — so no one can blame me for what happens. "Washing hands" is so prevalent and so widely accepted that we should not be surprised to find that doctors as well as officials in bureaucracies and institutions try to wash their hands of moral responsibilities when the going gets difficult.

There are, of course, situations in which "letting X happen," i.e., not preventing its happening, is commendable. Perhaps, indeed, such situations provide the rationale for some "washing hands." The most obvious examples of commendable abstinence are those involving interference in someone else's private affairs; it is a good idea not to intervene in a marital dispute, *to let* the couple say what they want to each other. The principle of non-intervention has a moral basis as well as a practical one, for it follows from the principle of respect for the liberty and moral autonomy of persons. The principle of self-determination, or liberty, is the opposite, of course, of paternalism, which holds that we have a right and a duty to make others do what *we* think is good for them, even if they do not agree with us. For example, it is paternalist to hold that *for his own good* it is right for us to force someone to stay alive even though he wants to die and thinks it the best thing for himself. The principle of "letting X happen" is therefore often a good antidote to paternalism, for, even though I know that what you plan to do will be disastrous, other things being equal, I have no right to prevent you from doing it. (Smoking is a good example; provided Jones's smoking is not a nuisance, does anyone have the right to prevent him from smoking? Shouldn't we just "let him smoke"? More controversially, does anyone have the right to prevent someone from committing suicide? Should someone have prevented Judas Iscariot from doing so?)

Let us see how these considerations about the morality of "letting X happen" apply to "letting a patient die." One might begin by asking: is letting this happen merely an escape, an abdication of responsibility, a washing of hands? or, on the other hand, is it an expression of respect for the moral autonomy of some person, say, the incurable, suffering patient? That is, is it a case of commendable non-intervention?

The medical issue is immensely complicated by the injection of mythology. Mythologists, especially theologians, often personify nature so that "letting X happen" is justified on the principle of non-intervention, e.g., letting nature take its course. On a theological level, we have statements like: only God has given life and only He can take it away. So "letting X happen" becomes a special case of non-intervention: namely, based on respect, *not* for the patient's will, but for Nature's or God's Will. It is assumed that, somehow, if we interfere with Nature, we are doing something analogous to interfering with a person's will. (It hardly seems necessary to dwell on the paradoxical side of this doctrine, which admits and encourages interference with and redirection of natural processes in almost everything else but the determination of the time of a person's death. At an earlier time, the notion that the coming of death was beyond human control — and was under the control of the gods might have made sense. But today, after all the things that we have done to upset nature, e.g., the processes of natural selection, it hardly seems consistent to insist on this one, miserable exception.)

Barring any further *proof* that God, if there is one, actually *intends* people to die in the agonizing way they do when one "lets them die," there is no reason why we ought to approve of letting an incurable, suffering patient die because of a principle of non-intervention that might be applicable, for example, to marital disputes and smoking. Nevertheless, the issues involved in non-intervention are very complicated and need to be discussed further.

First, we have to ask: *what* is being let (allowed) to happen? *What* is one refraining from preventing? What is it that one could prevent if one intervened? Sometimes a patient is allowed to die through termination of treatment; in that case one is refraining from prolonging his life. (As we shall see presently, one could ask why that is not killing him.) On the other hand, in letting a patient die, one is letting him suffer excruciating pain or letting him pass through a senile existence like a vegetable; then one is refraining from preventing suffering and a senile existence. If this is what is involved, letting him die would hardly seem commendable.

To pursue this point further, it should be noted that the notion of 'P's letting X happen' implies a counter-factual of the type: 'if P did Y, then X would not happen'. The question is then: what is Y? and how can P prevent X by doing Y? Omitting suffering, etc., that P could prevent, if X is the patient's death, then, *ex hypothesi* P cannot prevent X — in the long run, that is. All that P can do is to postpone X, the patient's death.

What I want to bring out here is that 'letting the patient die' is properly contrasted, logically, with 'treating the patient'. (Here we might restrict 'treatment' to life-prolonging treatment, excluding, for instance, palliation.) In a sense to be discussed presently, 'killing' and 'letting die' are not mutually exclusive alternatives. Hence, the question of the difference between them needs to be explored further.

Negative Acts

The question I now want to turn to is whether or not there is a significant ethical difference between doings and not-doings, performances and non-performances, or, in the jargon, between positive and negative acts. Is the not-doing of something subject to the same kind of moral standards used to judge and critically evaluate positive doings? Is refraining from treatment or letting a patient die significantly different logically and ethically from terminating treatment and hastening a patient's death, or killing him?

The intuitive view and that of the absolutist is that there is a significant difference, for, they hold, there is a significant difference between directly willing (or intending) an object and willing an object that, accidentally as it were, is the cause of something else. The principle involved here is known as the Principle of Double Effect.[17] An effect may be willed only if it is good, although the act leading to that good effect may also lead to an evil effect. Example: a doctor may perform an operation to save the baby of a pregnant mother (=good effect), even though the death of the mother is hastened thereby (=bad effect). The application of the principle has some strange and questionable consequences; for example, the bombing of a city is permissible if the aim is to destroy military targets even though civilian population are killed, but it is impermissible to kill civilian population *in order* to destroy military targets. From a moral point of view, it seems to me that the principle of double effect permits actions that are clearly wrong and prohibits actions that are clearly right. (This has been discussed elsewhere.)[18] In any case, the crucial difference lies not in the end-result but in the intention, the direct object of the will.

Without entering into a detailed discussion of the Thomistic theory of action that is involved here, suffice it to say that the conception of responsibility that it implies does not coincide with our ordinary notions of responsibility. As Casey shows, clearly and convincingly, we hold persons responsible for the consequences of their non-acts as much as for the consequences of their acts,[19] and that, of course, applies to the consequences of "indirect objects" of will as well as for those of its direct objects. (See my earlier remarks on negligence). Therefore a doctor is, other things being equal, as responsible for the consequences of non-treatment or letting a patient die as he would be for inducing his death directly. The indirectness of the act or its non-intentionality does nothing to relieve a person of his responsibility in the sense of what he ought to do. (It may, of course, provide extenuating circumstances mitigating culpability or blameworthiness — but that is an entirely different matter.) I would hold that a man who does something with good intention knowing that his act will also have evil consequences is just as much responsible for those evil consequences as he is for the good consequences that he intends. Only if we assume this to be true will we be able to explain why a person is often required to make amends or to repair the damage he causes knowingly in pursuit of a good cause. Goodness of intention is neither necessary nor sufficient to a person's being responsible for a state of affairs brought about his acts.

Leaving aside considerations about consequences, i.e. the value of possible states of affairs produced by a possible action as opposed to a possible non-action, we can still ask whether or not there is any significant difference between, say, attributing an action to a person and attributing a non-action to him. Is refraining from treating a person or permitting a disease to take its 'natural' course an action? Is refraining from telling the truth an action? Indeed, are all the possible acts that I am not now performing actions? As we shall see, this question essentially amounts to asking whether or not non-actions are a species of action. That is, does a non-action, e.g., refraining from doing something, possess all the ethically essential properties of an action? Can we ask the same kind of questions about non-actions?

The question is more complicated than it might at first appear to be. To begin with, we might want to distinguish between non-actions that are intentional or deliberately decided on and those that are not. It might be contended that deliberate non-actions partake of some of the features of positive actions because they involve the performance of a positive act of some kind, say, an act of deciding. Indeed, one can often take positive measures to avoid performing an act, e.g., one can avoid doing something by walking away or by hanging up on the telephone. In such cases, one might say that a person is accountable for deciding not to do A, or for doing some B in order to avoid doing A, but not accountable for not doing A. In that way, the "immaculateness" of a non-action might be preserved. I do not believe that this strategem will work, however, for reasons that I shall give shortly.

Again, the notion that non-actions are not actions may receive some support from the causal theory of action, that is, the theory that an action consists in a "causing something to happen," a "bringing about of something," etc.[20] Under this analysis, a non-action would presumably be a not-causing something to happen and, as such, would (by definition) not be an action. In other words, the causal theory of action seems to imply that we can only act positively (in the sense of *causing* something to happen). The omission of an act, a non-performance, would therefore not be an action, because it is a not-causing. If we add thereto a causal theory of responsibility, namely, the proposition that a person is responsible only for what he causes, then it follows that we are not responsible for our non-actions or, for that matter, for states of affairs we might have prevented.

Apart from the question of whether or not such a theory is philosophically acceptable, perhaps I have painted a philosophical caricature, something like it provides a kind of metaphysical underpinning for the washing hands attitude mentioned earlier; and it may explain why doctors feel more comfortable in not initiating treatment (not causing something to happen) than in terminating treatment (causing something not to happen). The question is whether or not a positive theory of action and of responsibility like this stands up.[21] For many obvious reasons, it would seem that it does not; for example, any acceptable theory of "responsibility" (in this sense), would have to accommodate counter-factuals, i.e. prpositions about what a person might have done (caused), if he had chosen.[22]

Accordingly, a consequentialist is quick to point out that responsibility is a function not only of what a person causes but of what he is able to cause and able to prevent, that is, it is a function of his *ability* to intervene in the causal nexus and influence the course of events. That this must be so, he would say, is necessary in order to be able to evaluate a certain outcome comparatively, by comparing it with other possible alternatives: a consequentialist must be able to compare actual consequences with possible consequences. Given the concept of counterfactual possibility, a consequentialist like Bennett,[23] for instance, can proceed to distinguish between 'killing' and 'letting die' in terms of "the only set of movements which *would* have produced that upshot" and "movements other than the only set which *would* have produced that upshot." In other words, 'to kill X' means that there is hardly anything else that one could do that would have the effect that the X dies and 'to let X die' means that almost anything that one could do would have the effect that X dies.

There are many reasons for rejecting this kind of analysis, however. For example, as Casey points out, a casual-counter factual analysis of this type includes many things that we would not ordinarily consider 'omission', 'refraining from doing,' or 'letting something happen'. The analysis is too broad and fails to capture important moral distinctions. There are limits to the kind of possible non-acts that we attribute to a person. Casey writes: "The view we take of a man's character, or of his role in a certain type of situation, sets limits not only on what we can regard him as responsible for in that situation but also, as we have seen, on what we can properly describe him as doing or refraining from doing."[24] There must be some reason to believe that the person in question is, or should be, *concerned* with what is happening. In his role as doctor, a person might be expected to treat or not to treat, but not to expend a thousand dollars from his private bank account to buy a drug for a patient that is needed to save her life.[25]

If we consider all the things that a person might do at a certain time *t*; let us call these possible acts PA's for X at t. Under normal circumstances, there is obviously an indefinitely large number of PA's for any person at any one time; he can wiggle his right middle toe, walk down the street differently — at a different speed, tread on a crack in the sidewalk, step on an ant, use different words or a different word-order in speaking, etc., etc. Certainly it would be absurd to say of most of these PA's that the person in question *failed*, refrained from or omitted to perform them. For most of them are outside the compass of meaningful consideration; we would not blame or commend a person for not-doing them, we do not deliberate about all the enormous number of PA's available, etc. In a sense, therefore, it is correct to say that it would be absurd to hold a person responsible for not doing a PA, as such. The term 'responsibility', in the sense involving possible blame or commendation, is inapplicable here. (I am not responsible for not wiggling my toe at 11:34 a.m. today, although I could have done so.)

Here again, one might ask: isn't not treating a patient such a non-act, such a neutral PA? If one could be held responsible for not performing PA's in general, would not a doctor who refrained from treating a terminal patient be simply refraining from performing one of those numerous PA's for which the notion of responsibility is irrelevant? His non-treatment, in that case, would as such be neither commendable or blameable, it would be completely neutral.

Our task is now clear: we must find some way or other of distinguishing between those PA's that are irrelevant to the assessment of conduct and those that are relevant. In our previous terminology, we need a way of determining whether a non-performance, a negative act, is an action or whether it is simply a PA which does not fall under the rubric of action at all and to which moral categories are inapplicable. There are two ways in which this can be done, I believe. The first involves the Why? of an action (accountability), and the second involves the What? and How? of an action (the structure of an act).

First, let us begin with the concept of an action in general. Here, borrowing from Ascombe, we might say that an action is the kind of thing regarding which one can ask for a reason. "Why did you do that?" [26] This logical property of actions will be called "accountability," by which I mean that it always makes sense to ask for an "account" of why one does or did something. (I use the term 'accountability' in order to distinguish what is involved here from other senses of the term 'responsibility'.)

Now, it should be clear that we often can and do ask for a person to account for his non-actions in the same way as one does for his actions. "Why didn't you do that?" "Why didn't you come?" "Why didn't you treat the patient?" The request for reasons of this type also arise in connection with propositions about what one ought to do: "Why shouldn't you refrain from treating?" "Why shouldn't you let the patient die?" and so on. In contrast, PA's that are not actions do not involve accountability in this sense: there are lots of things that I might do and it would be absurd to ask: "Why didn't you do that?" "Why didn't you wiggle your toe at 11:34 a.m. today?" "Why don't you step on the crack?" etc. The only way one could answer questions like that is to say: "I don't know. I never thought of it. Why do you ask? (i.e., why is it relevant?)" That is not to say, of course, that some of these irrelevant PA's might not become relevant through changing circumstances or once one attends to them.

The point that I want to emphasize is that many forms of non-action, refrainings and omissions, have the usual logical properties of actions, i.e., doings. This point is important because the simple not doing of something does not mean that one is "let off the hook"; one has to explain. A doctor who fails to treat ought to be able to give a reason for not-treating; in most cases, I am sure that this is possible. The hang-up is more likely to be philosophical than practical!

A second way of explaining the difference between PA's in general and non-actions (omissions) that are also actions is to see how the latter fit into the structure of action. Here we are concerned with questions like: "*What* are you doing?" or "*What* did he do?", on the one hand, and questions like: "*How* did he do it?", on the other hand.

It has now become a philosophical commonplace that the structure of an action is complex. One way of putting this is to say that one and the same act can be described in many different ways: Thus, Davidson writes:

"I flip the switch, turn on the light, and illuminate the room.

> Unbeknownst to me I also alert a prowler to the fact that I am at home. Here I do not four things, but only one, of which four descriptions have been given." [27]

Goldman, for reasons that it is unnecessary to enter into here, prefers to say that there are four different acts which are connected by the relation of "generation" in an act-tree. This relationship may be illustrated by saying, with regard to Davidson's example, that I illuminate the room by turning on the light, and I turn on the light by flipping the switch. The "higher level" acts are performed by (or in) performing "lower level" acts. The lower level acts generate higher level acts. Goldman offers a very useful analysis of the ways in which one act generates another.[28] The whole framework of acts thus generated from, e.g., one act, constitutes what he calls an act-tree. What Davidson and others call a single action (doing) with different descriptions amounts in Goldman's terms, to an act-tree made up of acts related to one another by "generation."

Because Goldman's detailed analysis is more helpful for us in the present discussion, I shall use his terminology rather than Davidson's. I should like to emphasize, however, that, as Davidson points out, there is a sense in which a person is doing one thing in doing many different things and vice versa. 'Treating', for example, has a set of complicated relationships to acts that generate it and to acts generated by it.

Now, one of the things that Goldman's analysis makes perfectly clear is that negative acts can be used to generate positive acts; that is, it is possible to do something by not doing something else. A driver can run over someone by failing to stop (by not-stopping); and a doctor can let his patient die by not treating him. Here, 'not treating' generates 'letting the patient die'. 'Letting him die' in turn might generate 'killing him', providing, of course, that we are able to explain how the doctor 'killed the patient' by (or in) 'letting him die'. If we add an intervening premise such as 'he let the patient die by starving him', to say that by these acts the doctor killed the patient becomes at least an intelligible statement.

The general lesson from all these theories of action is that doing one kind of thing does not automatically eo ipso exclude doing something else as well, that is, the appropriateness of one description of an action does not *eo ipso* entail the inappropriateness of another description. The conception that there is only one correct answer to the question: what is he doing? (or, what did he do? etc.) may be called the *fallacy of simple description*. It is obvious that this fallacy is often employed as a sophistic device to "get oneself off the hook." Thus, a person can plead: "I was just following orders" or, like Eichmann, "I was just organizing railroad schedules," or "I was just saving the baby," or "I didn't kill her, I just let her die." All such descriptions of particular acts are perfectly accurate, but they are clearly incomplete; for in all of them, there are other descriptions of the same action (or other acts on the act-tree) that are ethically more significant. It may be true that Jones pressed his fingers, thereby pulled the trigger and fired the gun, but it does not follow that Jones didn't kill the man! (We cannot say that the bullet killed him but not Jones!) [29] That the fallacy of simple description is a fallacy should be clear from the fact that many of the acts on this kind of act-tree are acts for which one is accountable; it makes perfectly good sense with regard to these acts to ask: why did you do that? One can ask of Jones, for instance, why did you press your finger? why did you pull the trigger? why did you fire the gun? and why did you kill the man? It should be observed that all sorts of answers are logically possible to such questions, ranging from excuses to justifications, as well as a simple: "I don't know." The point is, however, that such questions can be asked meaningfully — they are not odd or absurd.

There are two further points that have to be made in connection with the structure of action just discussed. The first point is that the selection of an act-description, or the construction of an act-tree, is not an arbitrary, subjective matter. It is not capricious, for, excluding metaphorical uses of language, there are built-in limits as to how an act can be described or generated. Goldman, for instance, examines in detail some of the methods of generation. According to his account, in general, an act A generates an act A', whenever there exists a set of generating conditions (C*) such that the conjunction of A and C* entail A'.[30] What this means, in effect, is that anyone linking two particular acts by

generation must be prepared to justify his doing so, that is, give ↑
reasons for saying, e.g., that 'Jones' letting Smith die' generates
'Jones killed Smith'. Since generating conditions often involve
reference to causality, the procedure of generation usually relates to specific instances rather than act-types. Hence generali-
zations in this area are apt to be deceptive.

In sum, anyone maintaining that there is a significant difference between not starting to treat a patient and terminating the
treatment of a similarly situated patient must show that the acts
generated by these two acts are significantly different ethically.
Thus, under certain circumstances, failing to turn on the
machine may in fact generate the same type of act as turning the
machine off, namely, they are both acts of 'letting the patient
die'. I will leave it up to the reader to apply the same line of
reasoning to some of the other situations discussed in this paper.

The second point concerns the bearing of act-descriptions,
act-generations and, in general, act-classifications on ethical
issues. One is tempted to say that some of them relate to essential
and others to accidental features of an action. For example,
whether Jones used his middle or his forefinger to press the
trigger is immaterial, what is essential is that he killed the man.
Bringing in the concept of essence at this juncture may appear to
confuse the issue. How does one determine what is essential and
what is accidental in an act? The intention? The consequences
for others in suffering? What accords with the essence or nature
of man?

It appears that we are now confronted with the doctrine generally known as "essentialism," the doctrine that there are
built-in essences of things and that it is up to us, as rational
beings, to determine what these essences are. Without entering
into a full-scale discussion of metaphysical essentialism, suffice
it to say that we are concerned here with what is essential from
the ethical point of view. If one is a consequentialist (or
utilitarian), one will take one view of what is essential; if one is
an absolutist (of the Thomistic variety), one will take another
view of what is essential. If one holds, as I do, that the social
relations between individual persons constitute the basic category of morality, then one will take even another view of what is
essential.

According to the ethics of the last type, integrity (e.g., telling the truth), understanding, helping, healing, relieving suffering, compassion, solicitude, and sympathy, along with their opposites, provide the context of acts that are ethically significant. And so those acts on the act-tree (or act-descriptions) that come under these categories are the ones with which we must be concerned in our medical decisions, as in other practical decisions.

A final word on killing. Killing, according to our analysis, can appear in a number of ways on an act-tree. One can kill another by driving dangerously, by shooting him, by depriving him of food, medicine or treatment, by operating on another person (as in Bennett's example), by executing him, etc. These are all act-types that usually generate killing. But killing itself can generate other acts, acts done by (or in) killing, e.g., freeing a prisoner, saving someone else's life, preventing a hold-up, depriving a family of its loved ones, making someone unhappy, ending unendurable suffering, etc. It is impossible to understand, much less to evaluate ethically, the act of killing apart from the other acts related to it in the act-tree — unless one holds that killing is itself an ethical category and that killing in itself is always wrong.

We now come to the final issue, namely, whether or not killing is, of itself, other things being equal, unconditionally wrong. Roman Catholic theologians generally take the position that the intentional taking of the life of an innocent human being is absolutely wrong. There are many ways in which this absolute principle is qualified, e.g. through the use of the principle of double-effect and a very flexible notion of what is to be included under 'innocence'. (It is all right to burn heretics and to kill the enemy in a war, for they are not "innocent.")

Nevertheless, with regard to killing, the *Onus Probandi* Principle requires us, as it does for other wrongful acts, to provide some reason why it is wrong. It will not suffice to show that killing is sometimes wrong, for that is easy. What is required is some sort of proof that killing is always wrong (except for the exceptions noted above). To say that euthanasia is wrong because killing is wrong is hardly an argument! Here we find no very convincing arguments.

It might be argued, for instance, that killing is taking away someone's life and life is always is a good in itself; therefore to kill is to destroy something that is good in itself. But leaving aside doubtful metaphysical and theological arguments, it is not at all obvious that life, in the biological sense, has any value other than instrumental. For any individual life (and health, for that matter) is a necessary condition of the pursuit, attainment and continuance of almost every good, including moral goods such as virtue and freedom. But that fact does not make life intrinsically good. Kant himself acknowledges this when he says in his discussion of suicide: "Life is not to be highly regarded for its own sake. . . . There is much in the world far more important than life. . . . The preservation of one's life is, therefore, not the highest duty."

The kind of life that is at issue in many cases of euthanasia is life in a quite minimal sense; often it is mere bodily existence without the possibility of any meaningful communication with others and consequently without the possibility of any meaningful moral relationship with them. If life is valuable as a condition of morality (or happiness), then it entirely loses its value when morality (or happiness) becomes impossible. By the same token, when, e.g., a body can no longer be the object of human concern, it loses its value. And so on through all the various positive (and good) arguments for preserving life.

According to the *Onus Probandi* Principle, if no more can be said in defense of the 'sanctity of life' under these minimal, perhaps even questionable conditions, then such life must be assumed to be morally neutral. Consequently, unless there are other reasons for not killing a minimally alive human body, then according to the Onus Probandi Principle, such killing is morally neutral. This is not to say that other reasons might not be forthcoming to make such killing either right or wrong. If so, then each such reason must be scrutinized and evaluated on its own merits.

One reason that has frequently been advanced against killing, as in euthanasia, is the so-called "slippery slope" or "camel's nose" argument — that once one permits euthanasia of consenting adults, one is led step by step until it is finally permitted for healthy, unconsenting adults who are classified as undesirable.

The argument, in its various forms, has been so widely discussed and refuted through use of obvious counter-examples
that I can add little that is new along these lines.[33] One point that
is frequently missed, however, is that the argument is plausible
only on the assumption that no meaningful ethical distinction
can be drawn between the life, say, of a mature, active person
and the life of an incurable, bedridden, perhaps senile human
body leading a vegetable existence. The slippery slope argument could appeal only to someone with very little moral sensibility to significant moral distinctions, for only if one neglects or
ignores such distinctions is there a problem of "sliding" from
one category to another. One is reminded of the rich man who
says that we needn't worry about the poor because it is difficult
to know where to draw the line between being rich and being
poor.

Throughout this paper I have deliberately refrained from offering glib solutions to the complicated problems under discussion. My main purpose has been to explore some of the underlying philosophical issues behind the distinction between negative and positive euthanasia.[34] What I have tried to show is that
if anyone persists in invoking this distinction in moral argument, it is incumbent on him to answer a great many questions,
questions of different sorts, the answers to which may be quite
different in different contexts. If he is unable to answer these
questions satisfactorily, then the presumption must be that the
distinction, as he is using it, is an invalid one.[35]

NOTES

1. A brief survey of the legal situation may be found in David Hendin, *Death as a Fact of Life* (New York: Warner Paperback, 1974), ch. 3.
2. See Daniel C. Maguire, *Death By Choice* (New York: Doubleday, 1973), ch. 2: The laggardly state of the law.
3. It has been suggested that doctors have an unusually strong fear of death and enter medicine as a counter-phobic defense against death. See Hendin, *op. cit.*, p. 115 for references.
4. See John Casey, "Actions and consequences," in John Casey, ed. *Morality and Moral Reasoning* (London: Methuen, 1971). I am indebted to Casey for many insights into the problem at hand.
5. St. Thomas Aquinas, *Summa Theologica*, IaIae, qu. 19, art. 9 ad 3.
6. See, for example, H. Davis, *Moral and Pastoral Theology*, 8th ed, ed. L.W. Geddes (London: Sheed and Ward, 1959), pp. 12-15.

7. "... it seems intuitively clear that causing a death is morally somewhat more reprehensible than knowingly refraining from altering conditions which are causing death." Daniel Dinello, "On killing and letting die," *Analysis* 31 (1971): 86.

8. For a good discussion of the Nazi argument, see Marvin Kohl, *The Morality of Killing* (New York: Humanities Press, 1974), especially p. 100.

9. See my *Ethical Relativism* (Belmont, California: Wadsworth, 1973), Introduction.

10. Kant, *Metaphysical Principles of Virtue*, tr. James Ellington (Indianapolis: Bobbs-Merrill, 1964), pp. 128-9. (Ak. Ausgabe, 463).

11. What I call moral neutrality is often called moral indifference. The argument presented here may also be found in "The Issue of Relativism," in *Ethical Relativism*, pp. 124 ff. It will be developed in more detail in a forthcoming book.

12. This is a typical ploy of destructive relativism. See note 11.

13. Indeed, the history of morals provides many illustrations of how some of the most strongly held convictions about morality have turned out to have a flimsy logical basis. For example, Victorian views on sex and primitive burial taboos.

14. The qualification "other things being equal" is necessary in order to exclude cases of compaative evils, for even the most rabid adherent of the principle that death is evil might admit that under certain circumstances it is a good, e.g. when someone dies to save the lives of others. The point that I am making relates to the contention that other things being equal, e.g. where there are no competing evils, death is an evil (i.e. an evil in itself). Socrates, on the other hand, held that death was a blessing, and he gave reasons why he thought it was so, just as he gave reasons why suicide was wrong. He did not invoke gut feelings or intuitions. See *Phaedo*, passim.

15. Thus parents were held guilty of 'involuntary manslaughter' and child abuse after they stopped insulin treatments for their child and he died. *Boston Globe*, July 20, 1974.

16. See my "Morality and the Ideal of Rationality in Formal Organizations," in *Monist* 54 (1970): 488-516.

17. See H. Davis, *op. cit..* (Note 6) and Joseph T. Mangan, "An historical analysis of the principle of double effect," *Theological Studies* 10 (March 1949): 41-61.

18. See my "Agressive War," presented at a symposium at Kane College, New Jersey, Spring 1974. To be published.

19. Casey, *op. cit.*

20. For a critique, see my "Ethical dimensions of the concept of action," *Journal of Philosophy* 62 (1965): 633-45. Also, Irving Thalberg, *Enigmas of Agency* (New York: Humanities Press, 1972), section 1. (References to literature on the causal theory may be found in Thalberg's book.)

21. For further arguments, see references in note 20.

22. I have enclosed 'responsibility' in quotation marks because I do not accept this use of the term. Strictly speaking, one can be responsible only for a state of affairs, not for actions. I have tried to develop a fuller theory of responsi-

bility in my "The Ethics of Participation,' in *Participation: Nomos XVI*, ed. Roland Pennock and John Chapman (New York: Atherton Press, 1975).

23. See Jonathan Bennett, "Whatever the Consequences." *Analysis* 26 (1966): 83-102.

24. Casey, *op. cit.*, p. 168.

25. Casey, *op. cit.*, p. 167.

26. See G.E.M. Anscombe, *Intention* (Oxford: Blackwell, 1957), p. 9.

27. Donald Davidson, "Actions, Reasons, and Causes," *Journal of Philosophy* 60 (1963). Reprinted in Norman S. Case and Charles Landesman, *Readings in the Theory of Action* (Bloomington: Indiana University Press, 1966), p. 180. See also, Alvin I. Goldman, *A Theory of Human Action* (Englewood Cliffs: Prentice-Hall, 1970).

28. Goldman, *op. cit.*, ch. 2.

29. It is obviously correct to say that the shooting, the bullet, Jones, etc., etc., killed him. One explanation does not exlude others. Sometimes it is said that the disease killed a patient rather than, say, a person. These are not mutually exclusive statements. Both might be true. Goldman, *op. cit.*, pp. 80 ff.

30. Goldman, *op. cit.*, p. 41.

31. A good critical discussion of 'innocence' in this connection is to be found in M. Kohl, *op. cit.*, ch. 3. and *passim*. Kohl points out the implication in many writings on the subject that death is a punishment and so only correctly inflicted on someone who is guilty.

32. Kant, *Lectures on Ethics*, tr. Louis Infield (New York: Harper Torchbooks, 1963), pp. 150, 152, 157.

33. For an illuminating discussion of the structure of this kind of argument, see Ch. Perelman and L. Olbrechts-Tyteca, *The New Rhetoric: a Treatise on Argumentation* (Notre Dame: University of Notre Dame Press, 1969) § 66: The Argument from Direction.

34. It should be clear by now why I prefer the terms 'negative and positive' to the more frequently used 'active and passive' euthanasia. The latter is a misnomer, because, as I have argued, by all the usual criteria, "letting a patient die" is no less an *action* than "killing him."

35. For an excellent discussion of the objectionable moral implications of the conventional doctrine that there is an important difference between these two kinds of euthanasia, see James Rachels, "Active and Passive Euthanasia," *New England Journal of Medicine* 292 (1975): 78-80. It seems more than likely that the true reason for the vehement opposition on the part of the medical profession to an objective re-examination of the distinction between "letting die" and "killing" is the profession's obvious vested interest in keeping the distinction alive. For once the distinction is abandoned, physicians will lose their present *de facto* monopoly over decision-making with regard to prolonging or terminating an incurable patient's life, a monopoly which they effectively exercise by custom and law in passive euthanasia. If the two categories of euthanasia are assimilated, then the decision to terminate will no longer be theirs; it will be made differently and on a different basis.

MICHAEL D. BAYLES

Euthanasia and the Quality of Life

The judgments and attitudes of many contemporary secular moral philosophers towards euthanasia diverge sharply from those of many enlightened leaders of society. Most people disapprove of euthanasia although they may not be willing to punish those who commit it — witness the tendency of juries to acquit in the rare instances in which trials are held. Leaders in the field of medical ethics usually approve allowing a patient to die, at least by withholding extraordinary treatment, but oppose intentional, direct killing of a dying patient even upon his request.[1] Yet, many philosophers are favorably disposed towards euthanasia in certain contexts.

There are three central issues with respect to the morality of euthanasia, defined as the intentional killing of another person from motives that include concern for his quality of life. (1) Is there a morally significant intrinsic difference between killing and allowing to die? (2) Is the consent of the patient necessary for euthanasia to be morally permissible? (3) What standards and criteria should be used to determine the value of continued life and thereby the rightness of euthanasia? When is life no longer worth living?

This paper focuses on the first and third of these issues. The issue of consent is too complicated to be adequately discussed here. However, there are certain types of cases, e.g., infants, in which consent of the patient is not possible. The first section of this paper argues that there is no intrinsic moral difference between killing and allowing to die. The second section examines the practical import of this conclusion with respect to euthanasia of consenting adults and infants. The final section discusses standards for evaluating the quality of life and criteria for judging the value of its continuation. Throughout, the discussion concerns the morality, not the legality, of euthanasia. The legal issue undoubtedly involves other considerations.

Killing versus Allowing to Die

John Ladd argues that ethics operates under the *Onus Probandi* Principle, that anyone who claims that one has a moral obligation to do or forbear from an action has the burden of proof to show why.[2] He thus places the burden of proof upon opponents of euthanasia. While one who claims that people have moral duties generally has the burden of proof, this interpretation of the *Onus Probandi* Principle does not work for all situations. The burden of proof is context dependent. In the context of moral dispute, someone who claims an exception to a mutually accepted moral rule or principle has the burden of proof. A more adequate interpretation of the *Onus Probandi* Principle is that one who claims a moral distinction has the burden of proof. The burden of proof thus falls upon those who claim there is a moral difference between allowing a patient to die and killing one. And if one assumes, as Ladd does, that most actions are morally permissible (or neutral), the burden of proof falls upon one who claims some actions are not permissible.[3]

Several points need to be clarified before particular arguments for a moral difference between killing and allowing to die may be examined. First, Ladd suggests that the distinction between killing and allowing to die is between withdrawing and withholding treatment, the former being a form of killing.[4] However, all major supporters of a moral difference classify withdrawal of treatment as allowing to die. The distinction is not between mere performance and non-performance. Moreover, whether a non-performance counts as an action is usually undisputed, because the non-performances in issue are intentional ones which almost everyone counts as responsible actions. Thus, developing a precise classification of those non-performances which count as actions attributable to a person does not significantly advance the argument.

Second, one must distinguish between various forms or kinds of treatment which may, however, be combined in one treatment regimen. One kind is treatment which cures a disease, e.g., antibiotics which usually cure pneumonia. Another kind of treatment does not cure a disease but sustains a patient's health by compensating for the disease and preventing debilitating effects, e.g., insulin for diabetes. Another kind of treatment neither cures nor compensates for a disease; instead, it retards the course of a disease, e.g., therapies which delay the progress of cancer or produce remissions. Yet another type of treatment merely sustains life, e.g., artificial respirators. The final kind of treatment simply alleviates symptoms, e.g., pain-killers and cough medicine.

The expression 'allowing to die' is sometimes used for this kind of symptomatic treatment — only caring for the dying. Herein 'allowing to die' does not mean this type of treatment although it does not exclude it; 'care' is used in the very restricted sense of such symptomatic treatment which does not prolong life (or does so only incidentally by reducing stress caused by symptoms). 'Allowing to die' is used to mean withholding or withdrawing treatment when it is probable that its institution or continuation would prolong a patient's life however briefly. It thus includes failure to provide cures, compensating treatments, disease-retarding therapies, and artificial life sustaining treatment.

Third, one must distinguish two forms of the claim that there is a moral difference between killing and allowing to die. One form holds that there is an intrinsic moral difference. Usually, it is held that there is an absolute duty not to kill but only a *prima facie* duty not to allow to die. However, it may be held that while both are only *prima facie* duties, the duty not to kill is stronger than that not to allow to die. Or, it may be held that there is a *prima facie* duty not to kill but no duty not to allow to die. Hence, even if there is an intrinsic moral difference, it need not always be dispositive of the overall moral evaluation of instances of killing and allowing to die. All of these versions agree that there is an intrinsic moral difference between killing and allowing to die which is always morally relevant. It always takes stronger reasons to justify killing (if it can be done at all) than it does to justify allowing to die. The second form of the claim that there is a moral difference between killing and allowing to die merely holds that *usually* there is a moral difference between the two. Hence, while usually there is a stronger duty not to kill than to allow to die, in some cases there is not. This form of the claim is a generalization from particular cases evaluated by considerations extrinsic to a difference between killing and allowing to die. The following discussion concerns only the first, not this second, form of the claim.[5]

To establish an intrinsic moral difference between killing and allowing to die, two conditions must be shown. (1) A logical or intrinsic difference must be shown between the two. (2) This difference must be shown to be morally significant. Ladd's argument against the distinction appears to be aimed at the first point, for he suggests that 'letting him die' might generate 'killing him'.[6] His example of this generation, letting the patient die by starving him, is not persuasive. Supporters of the distinction may argue that 'starving' is ambiguous between 'failing to provide food' and 'actively preventing from obtaining food.' If the latter is meant, then one has not "let the person die" but 'killed him'; while if the former is meant, one has 'let the patient die' but not 'killed him.' Moreover, as certain facts in addition to having 'let the patient die' are necessary to generate 'killed him,' the two are logically distinct. Finally, even if both descriptions may apply to "one act," it does not follow that no moral difference may be found. One may simply claim that when both apply, the duty not to kill is the more significant although one may violate two duties — not to kill and not to let die (if there is such a duty). In short, duties may be attached to descriptions of actions; and if two or more descriptions apply, one may have duties (or a duty and no duty) *qua* each description.

Five different grounds may be suggested for an intrinsic moral difference between killing and allowing to die. Each of them is frequently used in moral discussions. They are (1) the doctrine of double effect, and the distinctions between (2) actions and their consequences, (3) commissions and omissions, (4) sufficient and necessary conditions, and (5) positive and negative duties. Grounds (1) and (2) fail both to correlate with the difference between killing and allowing to die and to establish its moral significance. Grounds (3) and (4) fail to be morally significant, while ground (5) fails to correlate with the difference although it may be morally significant.

The doctrine of double effect permits performing actions which have a bad or evil effect that normally ought not be produced. The doctrine can be stated as follows: An action having both a good and a bad effect is permissible if (1) the bad effect is not intended as an end or means, and (2) the good effect outweighs the bad.[7] This definition needs to be clarified in several respects. First, it is assumed that the person knows the bad effect will occur. No moral consideration can be made if the bad effect is an unknown consequence, e.g., an unexpected effect of an experimental drug. Second, while the bad effect is known to occur, it is not intended as a conscious object of the action. Instead, the good effect is the conscious object. Third, since the bad effect cannot be intended as a means, it must be a known but unintended side effect.

The doctrine of double effect does not always distinguish between killing and allowing to die, nor is it morally acceptable. For example, suppose a physician withholds a life-prolonging treatment in order to bring about the early death of a patient and thus relieve his suffering. Since the physician intends the early death of the patient to end his suffering, he intends the patient's death as a means and the doctrine of double effect does not permit it. Essentially, the doctrine of double effect distinguishes between direct and indirect killing, not between killing and allowing to die. Moreover, the doctrine is not morally acceptable. Suppose both a woman and her unborn child will die unless she has an abortion, but the only possible procedure for the abortion involves intentionally killing the fetus. The doctrine of double effect does not permit the abortion even though the fetus will die whatever is done. In short, when a person will die whatever is done, the doctrine of double effect forbids deliberately hastening that person's death by killing as a means to saving the lives of others, no matter how many. A correct morality canot be so impervious to consquences.

The intentions of an actor may be relevant to distinguishing an action from its consequences. When one intentionally produces the death of a person, then the person's death is part of the action. When one does not intend the death of a person but merely foresees it, the person's death may not be part of the action but a (mere) consequence of it. This distinction between an action and its consequences is not identical to either the distinctions between killing and allowing to die or between direct and indirect killing. As construed, the consequences of an action may include either indirect killing or allowing to die. However, it is worth considering whether the distinction is morally significant, because if it is, there is a moral difference between direct killing and allowing to die.

Jonathan Bennett has penetratingly considered whether the difference between an action and its consequences is always morally significant.[8] While not disputing the distinction, he contends that there is no moral significance always (intrinsically) attached to it. Bennett shows that several features which might be thought relevant to the difference will not suffice. He frames his discussion in terms of the following example: A woman in labor will die unless an abortion involving a craniotomy is performed. If the abortion is not performed, then the fetus can be safely delivered. Performing the operation involves directly killing the fetus, but not performing it involves allowing the mother to die. If there is a moral difference between killing and allowing to die, then assuming the fetus and mother have equal rights, it is wrong to perform the abortion.

Consideration of this example shows that the action/ consequence distinction will not support a moral difference between killing and allowing to die. Several features which may be morally relevant do not necessarily attend the distinction between an action and its consequences. For example, there is no difference in the expectation or inevitability of death whether the abortion is performed or not. Nor is there a difference in the ultimate aim; for in either case, the ultimate aim is not to kill the mother or the fetus.[9] Thus, the difference must, Bennett claims, lie either in the immediacy of death upon the physician's movements or the difference between doing and refraining from doing. Under the concept of immediacy, Bennett includes a number of factors such as temporal or spatial proximity and complexity of causal connection. None of these factors is morally relevant. Philosophers generally agree that no preference is to be given for the temporal proximity of events. Nor is there any obvious reason why spatial proximity between movements and effects should count any more than temporal proximity. The same applies to the complexity of the causal connections. These factors may make a difference in the certainty of the outcome, but when the effects are known to occur in either case, these differences do not have any moral significance. With these other factors shown to be irrelevant, the only difference left is that between doing and refraining from doing. But that is precisely the point at issue here, so the distinction between actions and consequences could not support that point even if it did correlate with it.

Before considering other grounds for an intrinsic moral difference between killing and allowing to die, it is useful to follow Philippa Foot and distinguish two senses of 'allow'.[10] In one sense, to allow something is to enable it to happen. For example, one pulls the plug in the tub and allows the water to drain. In another sense, one allows something to happen by not interfering. These two senses are closely related, for the first is ceasing to prevent while the second is not preventing. Moreover, they correspond to the two types of situations usually referred to as allowing a patient to die. The first sense, ceasing to prevent, corresponds to withdrawing treatment, while the second sense corresponds to withholding treatment.

Several writers consider the distinction between killing and allowing to die to be a distinction between commissions and omissions. Foot suggests that the second sense of 'allow' requires an omission. Moreover, George Fletcher has claimed that for legal purposes the first sense should also be considered an omission. It is sufficient for classifying conduct as an omission, he claims, if people would describe it as permitting harm rather than causing it.[11] Since withdrawing treatment permits harm, it is an omission. If both senses of 'allow' involve omissions rather than commissions, then the distinction between commissions and omissions does correspond to that between killing and allowing to die.[12]

However, the distinction between commissions and omissions does not provide a basis for an intrinsic moral difference between killing and allowing to die. First, as von Wright has satisfactorily shown, there is no logical difference between the consequences of acts (commissions) and forbearances (omissions).[13] Second, in order to classify withdrawal of treatment as an omission, Fletcher argues that it merely permits (allows) the event (death) to occur. If the basis of a distinction between commissions and omissions is between causing death (killing) and permitting (allowing) it, then it cannot in turn be used to support a moral difference between killing and allowing to die. Third, one is morally responsible for omissions if one has a duty to act. Since a moral difference between commissions and omissions depends upon one's duties, one cannot use the distinction to support there being no duty or a lesser one to provide treatment in the case of omissions.

The distinction between the two senses of 'allow' may suggest another ground for morally differentiating killing and allowing to die. The notion of nonintervention involved in allowing to die presupposes an ongoing process which will result in death. Allowing a person to die of cancer implies a process which will result in the patient's death unless something is done. Forbearance from intervention is a necessary but not sufficient condition for death. Killing a person, however, does not presuppose an ongoing process which will bring about death. Instead, the action in killing a person is, in any situation, a sufficient, not a necessary, condition for the person's death. ('Killing', being a success word, logically entails death. 'Attempting to kill' does not logically entail death, but it merely brings in the element of certainty which has already been shown to be insufficient to establish an intrinsic moral difference between killing and allowing to die. Hence, 'the action in killing' is used to suggest that the logical connection is not intended and yet ignores the issue of certainty.) Thus, there is a "causal" difference between killing a person and allowing one to die. The action in killing is a sufficient condition for a person's death, but nonintervention (allowing to die) is only a necessary, not a sufficient, condition for a person's death.[14]

Nonetheless, this difference between necessary and sufficient conditions does not support an intrinsic moral difference between killing and allowing to die. People are generally held responsible for providing necessary as well as sufficient conditions for events. For legal responsibility, one does not usually require conduct to be a sufficient condition although it will suffice. The usual requirement is that the conduct be *sine qua non* for the result. Not everything which is a necessary condition for a result establishes causal responsibility in legal contexts, but in almost every instance in the particular situation the conduct is necessary for the event.[15] Since in the relevant sorts of situations a physician's not providing life-prolonging treatment is necessary for the death of the patient (at least sooner than would otherwise be the case), there is no reason on that ground for removing responsibility or claiming a moral difference between allowing to die and killing.

David Meyers has suggested a variation of the distinction between necessary and sufficient conditions for death. In the context of terminating extraordinary treatment, he distinguishes between causing the patient's death and not prolonging his death. The difference lies in the likely effects of the treatment, whether it preserves the patient's life and improves his living conditions or merely maintains certain bodily functions that have no independent viability without hope of improving his living conditions. If a physician terminates treatment in the latter situation, he does not cause the patient's death, "for it would already have come and claimed his patient *but for* the treatment being ceased."[16]

However, this distinction fares worse than the previous one. First, even with ordinary treatment, e.g., antibiotics for pneumonia, frequently the patient would already be dead *but for* the treatment. This factor holds for any life-prolonging or saving treatment. Second, Meyers rests much of the difference upon whether the patient can be restored to health. While such a consideration is obviously relevant, it has nothing to do with the distinction between killing and allowing to die. Instead, it concerns the prognosis and the physician's duties. Hence, if there is an intrinsic moral difference between killing and allowing to die, it must be found in a difference between the duties to treat and not to kill.

Foot believes that there is a significant difference in these duties which supports a moral difference between killing and allowing to die. She distinguishes between positive and negative duties. Roughly, negative duties are not to injure a person while positive duties are to benefit a person.[17] Negative duties are more basic or stronger than positive ones. Killing involves injuring or harming a person, whereas allowing to die is not benefiting a person. Since there is a stronger obligation not to injure a person than there is to benefit one, there is a stronger obligation not to kill a person than there is not to allow one to die.

This distinction between negative and positive duties obviously has some general appeal. It is wrong to steal $5000 from a person, but not to fail to give him $5000. Nonetheless, the distinction is incapable of bearing the significance Foot attaches to it. First, it is sometimes quite difficult to distinguish between nonbenefit and injury. Moreover, it raises the issue of who ultimately judges that something is a nonbenefit or injury — the patient, his family, or the physician. However, that issue may be ignored for now.

The second and more crucial point is that the judgments to support an intrinsic moral difference between killing and allowing to die must be such that killing always involves injury and allowing to die always involves nonbenefit. That is, killing must always violate a negative duty and allowing to die at most violate a positive duty. Foot does not retain the necessary correlations. She imagines not giving food to a beggar and allowing him to die so his body can be used for medical research. But, she comments, "presumably we are inclined to see this as a violation of negative rather than positive duty."[18] Consequently, as there are no strict correlations of negative duties with killing and positive duties with allowing to die, the distinction between negative and positive duties does not support an intrinsic moral difference between killing and allowing to die.

The upshot is that no intrinsic moral difference between killing and allowing to die has been established. Various proposed grounds for it have been examined — the doctrine of double effect and the distinctions between actions and consequences, commissions and omissions, necessary and sufficient conditions, and negative and positive duties. Consequently, various types of situations must be examined on their merits. Simplistic

moral thinking based upon an intrinsic difference is no more
satisfactory here than elsewhere. In the following section, the
practical import of this conclusion will be considered.

Unjustified Practices

The practical import of the conclusion that there is no intrinsic
moral difference between killing and allowing to die will be
considered with respect to two common practices. The first is
denying voluntary euthanasia to dying adult patients while
respecting their requests not to receive extraordinary life-
prolonging treatment. The second practice is allowing infants
with birth defects to die by withholding ordinary treatment.

Not everyone believes it is permissible to comply with the
wishes of an adult patient that he be allowed to die. Those who
deny that it is ever right to withhold or withdraw life-prolonging
or saving treatment agree that there is no intrinsic moral difference between killing and allowing be die. Consequently, only
those people who believe that in some situations it may be right
to allow a patient to die but not to kill him disagree with the
above conclusion. All of them agree that in some situations it is
permissible for a physician to comply with a patient's request to
be allowed to die by withholding extraordinary as opposed to
ordinary life-prolonging treatment. The distinction between extraordinary and ordinary life-prolonging treatment is subject to
much debate by physicians and moralists. For present purposes,
the precise nature of this distinction is irrelevant. The arguments below hold whenever treatment is classified as extraordinary. In general, extraordinary treatment may be taken as involving any medicine, operation, or equipment which is unusual
and expensive, painful, or otherwise very inconvenient.[19]

If it is right to comply with an adult patient's voluntary,
sincere request to be allowed to die by withholding or withdrawing extraordinary life-prolonging treatment, then the patient is
the ultimate judge of the value of the extra life which the treatment might provide. That it may only be right to comply with
such a request under certain circumstances, e.g., one believes
the patient can not live much longer anyway, does not negate
this point. Under whatever circumstances one wishes to define,

the patient's judgment is authoritative. Consequently, under similar circumstances the patient's judgment that he should die now must be accepted. That is, if under similar circumstances the patient voluntarily and sincerely requests that he be killed, then one must accept his judgment that whatever future life he might have left would be a burden to him rather than a benefit. Sometimes attempts are made to avoid this conclusion by the question-begging assertion that any patient who makes such a request *must be* incapable of rational choice.

If it is right to allow the patient to die in the one case, it is also right to kill him in the other because there is no intrinsic moral difference between killing and allowing to die. Indeed, since by hypothesis the patient's judgment is authoritative in the situation, to deny either request is wrong. It is morally equivalent to inflicting upon the patient the hardship which he undergoes during the time he lives but would not have undergone had one complied with his request. In short, in these circumstances not to comply with a patient's request for euthanasia (killing) is morally equivalent to inflicting on him as torture whatever he suffers the rest of his life.

A patient may rationally decide to forgo extraordinary life-prolonging treatment but not request to be killed. He may determine that while if given care his life is not such that he would prefer to die, neither is it of sufficient value to be prolonged. Or, he may judge that the extra life he would gain from an extraordinary life-prolonging procedure would come at the end when his condition would have so deteriorated that life would no longer be worth living even if given care. However, it is also possible that extraordinary life-prolonging treatment extends the time when, given care, life is of a quality worth living and the patient therefore requests it.

Perhaps in recognition of this symmetry between killing and allowing to die, arguments against voluntary euthanasia have emphasized untoward effects of a policy permitting voluntary euthanasia.[20] But these arguments also apply to allowing a patient to die by withholding or withdrawing extraordinary life-prolonging treatment. The three major ones will be briefly examined.

The first argument is the "wedge" argument. Essentially, it contends that permitting voluntary euthanasia would be to admit the thin edge of the wedge. Once voluntary euthanasia is permitted, there is no stopping short of killing all those whom society thinks are unfit or unhappy.[21] Logically, the argument is balderdash. F. M. Cornford described it as the principle "that you should not act justly now for fear of raising expectations that you may act still more justly in the future. . . ."[22] It might be made valid by adding an empirical premise that the undesired extensions will probably occur. However, a similar claim may be made concerning allowing to die by not using extraordinary means of life-prolongation. Without scientific studies supporting either claim, neither provides any basis for a conclusion against either practice. It would be worth investigating the point at which distinctions become too fine to be useful in moral rules. Nevertheless, it is implausible that ordinary people cannot distinguish between killing dying patients upon their request and killing relatively healthy persons without their consent.

A second argument, or set of arguments, rests upon uncertainty. A physician may misdiagnose as terminal an illness which is not. A cure may be found before the patient would otherwise have died. And it is difficult to establish that the patient does make a fully voluntary and sincere request that his life be ended. Indeed, this last point is sometimes turned into a certainty that the patient cannot voluntarily consent to having his life terminated because of pain, effects of drugs, etc. Surely this last ploy is taking the argument too far. However, no one is ever certain (in the sense sought) about empirical matters relevant to moral judgments. If a cancer patient has metastases throughout his body, one can be quite sure he will not live much longer. In any case, the very same points apply to allowing to die by not using extraordinary means of life-prolongation. The diagnosis might be mistaken, a cure might be found in the extra time provided, or the patient may object to its not being used. Mistake-proof medicine and morals are not human medicine and morals.

The final objection to be considered is that euthanasia would undermine the doctor-patient relationship. The patient would no longer trust his doctor not to "do him in." [23] This objection is plausible for compulsory euthanasia, but it applies equally to allowing patients to die without their consent. When both procedures are based on the wishes of the patient, there is little reason to believe that the relation of confidence will be undermined. Indeed, noncompliance with patients' wishes for euthanasia might well undermine the relationship more than compliance.

Consequently, the practice of complying with adult patients' requests to die by not having life-prolonging treatment but not complying with similarly circumstanced patients' requests for euthanasia is morally unjustified. The patients' judgments as to the value of their continued life must be respected equally in both situations. The arguments from untoward consequences of the practice of voluntary euthanasia apply equally well or poorly to the practice of not using extraordinary life-prolonging treatment. Finally, it is sometimes suggested that only a very few patients request to be killed. Even if true, that is certainly not a reason against its moral rightness. The moral rightness of an action does not depend upon the frequency of the occasion for it.

The second unjustified practice is allowing defective newborn infants to die by withholding or withdrawing what in at least some cases is ordinary treatment. There has recently come to public attention a number of cases where treatments which are usual for the disease or problem and likely to prolong life have been withheld or withdrawn from newborn infants.[24] Generally, in these cases the infant has two or more genetic or congenital defects, such as Down's syndrome (mongolism) and an obstruction or defect of the gastrointestinal tract. If the latter defect is not repaired by surgery, then the infant will soon die; if it is repaired, then the infant may live for an indefinite period of time — perhaps a number of years.

In several cases, the parents have refused to consent to the operation. Intravenous feeding, etc., have been discontinued and after a time the infant has died. In the famous Johns Hopkins case, the infant lingered fifteen days before dying. Some commentators believe that sometimes it is permissible not to provide the life-prolonging treatment but wrong to kill the infant. On what grounds one may decide not to "save" or prolong the life of such an infant is not in dispute at this point. What is in dispute is leaving the infant to a lingering death rather than killing it.

As there is no intrinsic moral difference between killing and allowing to die, once a decision is made in such cases not to prolong life, the infant should be killed. The decision not to prolong life implies *ceteris paribus*, a judgment that the future life the infant might have were the treatment given is not of sufficient quality to be worth living. Consequently, the extra time lived in allowing to die rather than killing is not worth living. While it may be rational for an adult to forgo life-prolonging treatment but not be killed because the period of life gained by the treatment might only come at the end when, despite care, life is not worth living, with infants such a judgment does not seem generally reasonable. The longer an infant lives, the more it will develop whatever limited capacities it may have. Hence, the latter part of its life is apt to be of higher, not lower, quality and so more worth living. The only plausible ground for a contrary judgment is that the infant, as it developed, would be more aware of its defects or pain and so suffer more. However, there is no reason to believe that an older infant is more conscious of physical pain than a newborn one. If it becomes more aware of its defects, then it might be killed at a later time. If the infant suffers sufficiently at the time to render further life not worth living, then in not killing it one merely inflicts further days of suffering upon it.

Moreover, there is an added burden on adults involved in not killing an infant. Those who decide not to treat may view the remaining life as one of suffering and thus suffer more themselves. Those who disagree with the decision will be upset by the sight or knowledge of the dying baby. This burden upon others is greater with infants than it is with adults upon whose request treatment is forgone. An adult has consented to die in such a fashion, so others may be comforted with the view that he is at least dying as he desires.

The case of such infants is empirically similar to that of injured animals. Newborn infants, unlike adults, have conscious capacities similar to animals. They are primarily restricted to consciousness of their physical state. If anything, newborn infants have less consciousness of their environment than do many adult mammals. Yet it would be deemed wantonly cruel, even criminal, to allow a fatally injured animal to die rather than kill it. This parallel with animals is frequently drawn in discussions of euthanasia, but it is most relevant in the case of infants. The stock (false) objection is that people are not animals. As Antony Flew has replied, "This is precisely not a ground for treating people worse than brute animals." [25]

The general point being made cuts both ways. As there is no intrinsic moral difference between killing and allowing to die, if it is wrong to kill a defective infant, it is as wrong to allow it to die by withholding life-prolonging treatment except for the small amount of extra life in the latter case. People cannot assuage their consciences by asserting that they did not kill an infant but only allowed it to die. Whatever the criteria as to when one should or should not prolong the life of infants, if there are sufficient reasons not to prolong an infant's life, then it ought to be killed; and if it is wrong to kill it, it is also wrong to allow it to die. In either case, allowing an infant to die is unjustified.

This section has not considered the substantive criteria as to when life may not be worth living or prolonging. Instead, it has been restricted to issues about how people die once a judgment is made or recognized that life is not worth prolonging. The final section considers grounds for judgments that a life is not worth living or prolonging.

Value of Life Judgments

As Hudson correctly points out, semantic and conceptual precision cannot be achieved as to quality of life. [26] However, the reason is not, as he suggests, the uniqueness of each biological situation. On the one hand, everything in the universe is unique in that it is different from everything else. On the other hand, biological situations are sufficiently similar for physicians to develop general practices and therapies of choice which apply to many people and situations. Rather, the difficulty is that the judgments require the application of standards which admit of degrees. But just as the legal standards of due care, fair rate, and good faith may be indisputably applied over a wide range of cases despite uncertainty in others, so likewise, allowing for their greater abstractness, may standards as to the quality and value of life.

While 'quality of life' is much in vogue, the expression is ambiguous. Different ethical theories provide different standards and criteria for evaluating the quality of life and whether it is worth living. In particular, utilitarian and perfectionist standards of quality of life are quite distinct. The rest of this section briefly sketches these standards and considers criteria using them in making judgments about the value of continued life.

The utilitarian standard of the quality of life is simply the net happiness (degree of happiness minus the degree of unhappiness) experienced at a moment.[27] The quality of life is good or has positive value as long as happiness exceeds unhappiness; it is bad when unhappiness exceeds happiness. Nonexistence is ascribed the same value as zero net happiness. In short, the quality of life at a moment is simply the overall happiness or unhappiness one then experiences.

There are two utilitarian criteria for evaluating the value of *life*. One criterion is to maximize the "total amount of happiness" in a life, which is simply the sum of the net happiness experienced during the time lived. (One must allow for variation in the quality of life over time.) This criterion has a common sense basis in the ideas that the more net happiness in a life, the better it is; and that as long as one is happy, the longer one lives the better. By this criterion, a life is not worth continuing when its total happiness will not be increased.

The other utilitarian criterion is to maximize the "average level of happiness" in a life which is simply the average of the quality of life at the various moments. For example, if one had a net happiness of two units at a moment for one week and four units for the next, the average level for the two weeks would be three units. The common sense basis of this criterion is that it is not the length of life which counts but how good it is while it lasts. It is better to live a shorter, more eventful, and intensely happy life than a long, relatively dull one of moderate happiness even if there is more total happiness in the latter. By this criterion, as long as the expectable level of happiness is as high as the average for one's previous life, it is worth living. When the rest of one's life is likely to involve a significantly lower average level of happiness, it is not worth living. This criterion thus allows for some decline from a peak level of happiness, but if in advancing years one's level of happiness declines permanently below the average of one's previous life, it is not worth continuing to live.

Perfectionist standards of quality of life provide the main alternatives to the utilitarian standard. Perfectionist standards specify certain qualities (activities and actualizations of capacities) which determine the quality of life. Generally, certain qualities or a minimum number are thought necessary for a quality of life worth living, and the more such qualities in addition to the minimum or necessary ones the higher the quality of life. Perfectionist standards vary depending upon the qualities specified. They are often closely tied to the concept of personhood, specifying qualities such as self-awareness, memory, love, communication, conceptual thinking, and physical mobility.[28] If a person has prospects for the development or continued use of the necessary or minimum number of qualities, his life is worth living. If he cannot have such qualities, then his life is not worth living even if it will involve positive net happiness. A varation or addition to perfectionist standards involves considerations of the overall coherence of a lie. Samuel Gorovitz's conception of a life as a biography, with appropriate and inappropriate possible endings, is an example of such a perfectionist criterion for evaluating a whole life.[29]

Dallas High correctly claims that attention should be paid to a dying patient's quality of life and the possibilities of providing care. But he misleadingly suggests that the choice between life prolongation, euthanasia, and allowing to die is a false issue.[30] If life-prolongation is possible, these alternatives are exhaustive; one either provides life-prolonging treatment or not, in which case one either allows the patient to die or kills him. High's valid point is that in choosing between these alternatives each must be evaluated on the assumption that care will be provided to maintain as high a quality of life as possible. However, one must not assume, as High appears to do, the context of advanced Western medicine. For most people of the earth, medical personnel, supplies, and facilities are simply not available to provide even the type of care High recommends. Of course, these conditions also obviate worries about drastic attempts to prolong life. The rest of this section considers when, given the best possible care, termination of life is appropriate on the different criteria for the value of continued life.

The specific factors for determining the quality of life are likely to be similar on the utilitarian and perfectionist standards, because the qualities included in the latter also usually increase happiness. In judging the quality and value of continued life, three types of specific factors are predominant: mental capacity, physical capacity, and pain. Proponents of euthanasia have usually emphasized pain as the primary factor indicating termination of life. Such an emphasis implies a utilitarian standard of quality of life. On a perfectionist standard, pain need not imply a quality of life not worth continuing unless it interferes unduly with other factors, e.g., impairs mental functioning. And as High suggests, it may now be possible to control pain in most cases.[31]

However, even in the absence of pain, mental or physical incapacity may indicate that life is no longer worth living. By the total happiness criterion, the incapacity must be such that there is negative net happiness. By perfectionist criteria, the incapacity need only be such that one no longer has the necessary or minimum number of qualities. For example, if one classifies physical mobility as necessary, then paralysis from the neck down may deprive one of a quality of life sufficient to make it worth living. Finally, by the average level of happiness criterion, one's life may no longer be worth living even though one has considerable mental and physical capacity. One's incapacity need only be such that the expectable average level of happiness for any subsequent period of life is below the average level to that time. Consequently, by any one of these criteria a patient free from pain may correctly judge that future life is not worth living.

In making a judgment to end one's life, one may also consider duties to others. Tristram Engelhardt argues that, because one is excused from most duties by incapacitation, duties to others do not usually present grounds for judging that a dying person ought to live longer.[32] But incapacity excuses only when it renders one incapable of fulfilling a duty; if one can obtain substitute performance, one is not excused. For example, an ill teacher may be able to get someone else to take over his classes. Moreover, one may have a duty not to impose a great burden on others. If so, and one's continued life would be a great burden on others, then one may have a duty to end it. Thus, one may properly judge that one's life should be ended, even though were it not for the burden it would place upon others it would be of sufficient quality to be worth living. As such a judgment needs to be made upon a realistic appraisal of the burden imposed on others, a patient should be frankly told about the financial and emotional burden being shouldered by his family or friends.

The differences between the criteria of the value of continued life are most marked when one must judge whether the lives of others are worth prolonging. When the other person is an adult, one should probably use the criterion that person would use. If one uses a different criterion, then one may terminate life which the patient would find worth living or extend life the patient finds not worth living. When, however, the other person is a newborn infant, one must decide which criterion is appropriate, and it need not be the same criterion one would use for one's own life.

The total happiness per life criterion rarely supports killing a defective infant or allowing it to die. The question is whether the infant experiences more happiness than unhappiness. If it does, then its life is worthwhile. The difficulty is in determining whether it experiences more happiness than unhappiness. However, if it suffers no or little pain (does not cry frequently, etc.), then as it has few other sources of unhappiness, its happiness is probably greater than its unhappiness.

The average level of happiness criterion is somewhat more difficult to use. Infants have little or no previous life to establish an average level of happiness. Moreover, as their life has been at such a primitive level, any significant development is likely to increase their level of happiness. For example, a week old infant with Down's syndrome is likely to develop enough mentally and physically to greatly increase its average level of happiness. Being retarded, it is not likely to experience anguish from a realization of its incapacity as compared to normal children.

At this point, it is tempting to use an interpersonal criterion of average level of happiness — is this infant likely to have an average level of happiness comparable to that of normal children? But this interpersonal criterion of average level of happiness is fatally defective. Applied to the normal population, it implies that the lives of all those below the average level of happiness in the society are not worth living. If all those lives which are not worth living are eliminated, then one has a new average level of happiness in society and another set of lives which are not worthwhile. By successive applications of the criterion and elimination of worthless lives, one may reduce a population to its happiest member (assuming the loss of the other lives would not decrease his happiness).

Perfectionist criteria are most likely to support a judgment that a defective infant's life is not worth prolonging. How many infants would be so judged and how defective they must be depends upon the qualities used in the standard of quality of life. But suppose, with minimal plausibility, that the necessary qualities for positive value are those required for living on one's own in society. Then any infant which does not have the potentiality of developing into a self-sufficient member of society does not have a sufficiently high expectable quality of life to make it worth living. Of course, this standard is pretty high, probably the highest a non-Nietzschean would set, but even lower standards may imply that the lives of many defective infants are not worth living.

This analysis has only considered whether an infant's life is worth living. A decision upon termination might take into account benefits or burdens of others. It is ethically questionable whether possible benefits or burdens of others should be considered. Considering benefits would make a difference only if one judged that the life in question was not in itself worth living but would benefit others. For example, on a high perfectionist standard of quality of life, the life of an infant with Down's syndrome might not be worth living, but it might bring considerable happiness to its parents. However, one would then be prolonging a worthless life for the benefit of others — using the infant as a mere means (because it does not benefit at all) to the ends of others. The same objection would arise if an infant's life would be worth living but terminated because it would be a burden to others.

This objection to considering the burdens and benefits of others arises only on a nonutilitarian ethical view, which is unlikely to use a utilitarian standard of quality of life. Utilitarians would consider the benefits and burdens of others. A crucial problem in considering burdens and benefits of others is the extent to which public monies are used to pay for medical care. If public monies are used, then the burdens of continuing an infant's life may be acceptable to its parents; but if they are not available, the combined financial and emotional strain might overwhelm a family. This issue cannot be pursued further here.[33]

It has thus been shown that there is no basis for an intrinsic moral difference between killing and allowing to die. Thus, the practices of honoring requests by adults not to receive extraordinary life-prolonging treatment while denying requests of similarly circumstanced adults for euthanasia and of allowing defective infants to die instead of killing them are morally unjustifiable. These practices take as given judgments about the value of prolonged life. There are at least two kinds of standards for evaluating the quality of life and various criteria for judging the value of its continuation. While the different criteria result in varying judgments as to when life is of sufficient quality to be worth living, they all support the claim that in some contexts life is no longer of value. Since benefits and burdens of others are not always significant, each criterion implies that sometimes a life is not worth prolonging. Consequently, euthanasia of dying adults and defective infants is morally justified in some contexts.

NOTES

1. House of Delegates of the American Medical Association, *Journal of the American Medical Association* 227 (1974): 728; Pope Pius XII, *New York Times*, 25 November 1957, p. 1; Edwin F. Healey, S.J., *Medical Ethics* (Chicago: Loyola University Press, 1956), pp. 67, 266; and Arthur J. Dyck, "An Alternative to the Ethic of Euthanasia," in *To Live and To Die: When, Why, and How*, ed. Robert H. Williams (New York: Springer-Verlag, 1973), p. 104. While it is not completely settled, this distinction also appears in the law: David W. Meyers, "The Legal Aspects of Medical Euthanasia," *BioScience* 23 (1973): 467-68; Survey, "Euthanasia: Criminal, Tort, Constitutional and Legislative Considerations," *Notre Dame Lawyer* 48 (1973): 1207-10, 1242-44; and George P. Fletcher, "Prolonging Life: Some Legal Considerations," in *Euthanasia and the Right to Death*, ed. A. B. Downing (New York: Humanities Press, 1970), pp. 75-76, 84 [hereinafter this book is cited as *Euthanasia*]. Moreover, it reflects physicians' attitudes: Diana Crane, "Physicians' Attitudes Toward the Treatment of Critically Ill Patients," *BioScience* 23 (1973): 472; Robert H. Williams, "Propagation, Modification, and Termination of Life: Contraception, Abortion, Suicide, Euthanasia," in *To Live and To Die*, pp. 90-91.

2. "Positive and Negative Euthanasia," in this volume, p. 110.

3. A complete analysis of the allocation of the burden of proof in arguments generally, and those about euthanasia in particular, would be much more complex than that given in the text.

4. Ladd, "Positive and Negative Euthanasia," pp. 107, 122.

5. A confusion between these two forms of the claim may be seen in the writing of Paul Ramsey. In a justly famous discussion of care of the dying, he at first asserts that the distinction between allowing to die and killing, which he treats as that between omissions and commissions, "must be taken into account" and "is of first importance." *The Patient as Person: Explorations in Medical Ethics* (New Haven: Yale University Press, 1970), pp. 118, 151. However, as the discussion proceeds, he considers it less important. Instead, he emphasizes providing care and suggests that as the treatment would be useless, withholding or withdrawing it is only incidentally not doing something (pp. 151, 159); it is primarily substituting care when life cannot be prolonged. Finally, he clearly makes the difference a generalization and not an intrinsic one, because if care for the dying should no longer be possible, as with a comatose patient, "the basic reason for a significant moral distinction between omission and commission is abrogated" (p. 162; see also p. 163). Thus, the difference between killing and allowing to die is not itself morally significant but rather which option may benefit the patient.

6. "Positive and Negative Euthanasia," p. 120.

7. Healey, *Medical Ethics*, p. 98; Norman St. John-Stevas, *Life, Death and the Law* (Cleveland: World Publishing Company, Meridian Books, 1961), p. 190; John C. Ford, S.J., "The Morality of Obliteration Bombing," in *War and Morality*, ed. Richard A. Wasserstrom (Belmont, Cal.: Wadsworth Publishing Company, 1970), p. 26. How one determines whether an effect is intended is a difficult issue but not relevant here.

8. "Whatever the Consequences," in *Moral Problems*, ed. James Rachels (New York: Harper & Row, 1971), pp. 42-66.

9. *Ibid.*, p. 48.

10. "The Problem of Abortion and the Doctrine of the Double Effect," in *Moral Problems, op. cit.*, pp. 35-36.

11. "Prolonging Life," pp. 77, 79.

12. Some physicians may believe there is a moral difference between withholding and withdrawing treatment, being less inclined to do the latter (Ramsey, *Patient as Person*, p. 121). The distinction between commissions and omissions does not support that difference since both withholding and withdrawing treatment are classified as omissions.

13. Georg Henrik von Wright, *Norm and Action: A Logical Enquiry* (London: Routledge & Kegan Paul, 1963), p. 48.

14. This analysis differs from that of Bennett. He claims that the only difference is that in killing, of all the movements a physician might perform, few result in death; while in allowing to die, of all the movements a physician might perform, almost all result in death. "Whatever the Consequences," pp. 57-58. The distinction in the text essentially agrees with that by Daniel Dinello, "On Killing and Letting Die," in *Ethics and Public Policy*, ed. Tom L. Beauchamp (Englewood Cliffs, N.J.: Prentice-Hall, 1975), p. 357. Dinello claims there is an intuitive moral difference, but his claim is open to Ladd's criticisms of relying on intuitions ("Positive and Negative Euthanasia," pp. 000-00.)

15. See generally, H. L. A. Hart and A. M. Honoré, *Causation in the Law* (Oxford: Clarendon Press, 1959), chap. 5. In The Queen v. Instan, [1893] 1 Q.B. 450, a woman was convicted of felonious homicide for failing to provide her aunt food and care which "substantially accelerated" death from exhaustion caused by gangrene.

16. "Legal Aspects," p. 469. There is a tendency for those who discuss such cases to assume the patient is already dead by brain death criteria. Meyers' example of not prolonging death is "cessation of mechanical respiration wherein cerebral hemorrhage has caused irreversible cessation of the patient's spontaneous brain function, assuming the latter to be a medically acceptable, conclusive criterion of death." See also Crane, "Physicians' Attitudes," p. 473. Such an assumption may be very misleading, for the dead can neither be killed nor allowed to die.

17. "Problem of Abortion," p. 37. See also W. D. Ross, *The Right and the Good* (Oxford: Clarendon Press, 1930), pp. 21-22.

18. "Problem of Abortion," p. 38. Michael Tooley suggests that the reason one is tempted to correlate negative and positive duties with killing and allowing to die concerns plausible motivational inferences and the effort involved in action as opposed to inaction; "Abortion and Infanticide,' *Philosophy & Public Affairs* 2 (1972): 59-60.

19. See Ramsey, *Patient as Person*, pp. 121-22; St. John-Stevas, *Life, Death and the Law*, p. 275; Healey, *Medical Ethics*, p. 67.

20. See Yale Kamisar, "Euthanasia Legislation: Some Non-Religious Objections," in *Euthanasia*, pp. 85-133; St. John-Stevas, *Life, Death and the Law*,

pp. 271-75; and Sissela Bok, "Euthanasia and the Case of the Dying," *BioScience* 23 (1973): 462-63.

21. See, for Example, James F. Toole, "The Concept of Brain Death as Viewed by a Neurologist," in this volume, p. 58; and Robert P. Hudson, "Death, Dying, and the Zealous Phase," in this volume, pp. 76-77.

22. Quoted in Paul A. Freund, *On Law and Justice* (Cambridge: Harvard University Press, Belknap Press, 1968), p. 55.

23. Hudson, "Death, Dying, and the Zealous Phase," p. 76. His claim that medical skills and judgment are needed for passive euthanasia (allowing to die) is surely false; it takes no medical skill *not* to administer treatment. What may require medical skill is providing care to a patient not receiving life-prolonging treatment.

24. See, for example, the cases discussed in David H. Smith, "On Letting Some Babies Die," *Hastings Center Studies* 2 (May 1974): 37-46; Richard A. McCormick, S.J., "To Save or Let Die: The Dilemma of Modern Medicine," *Journal of the American Medical Association* 229 (1974): 172-76; Anthony Shaw, "Dilemmas of 'Informed Consent' in Children," *New England Journal of Medicine* 289 (1973): 885-90; and Raymond S. Duff and A. G. M. Campbell, "Moral and Ethical Dilemmas in the Special-care Nursery," *New England Journal of Medicine* 289 (1973): 890-94.

25. 'The Principle of Euthanasia," in *Euthanasia*, p. 34.

26. "Death, Dying, and the Zealous Phase," pp. 68-71.

27. This discussion of the utilitarian standard and criteria has benefited from an unpublished paper by Lawrence N. Davis. He has shown how the standard and criteria for the value of a life may be given mathematical expression clearly indicating their differences.

28. See Hudson, "Death, Dying, and the Zealous Phase," p. 69.

29. "Dealing with Dying," in this volume, pp. 29-30.

30. "Quality of Life and Care of the Dying Person," in this volume, p. 88.

31. *Ibid.*, p. 101.

32. H. Tristram Engelhardt, Jr., "Rights and Responsibilities of Patients and Physicians," in this volume, p. 20.

33. I develop a principle for the appropriateness of using public monies for certain types of health care in "National Health Insurance and Noncovered Services," *Jounal of Health Politics, Policy and Law* 2 (Fall 1977).

ROBERT M. VEATCH

Natural Death and Public Policy

> *Thou shalt not kill; but need'st not*
> *strive officiously to keep alive.*

Strange world this. That a serious argument must be made that
death is an evil to be conquered. That now when for the first time
in human history we have the power to conquer at least some
deaths, we should begin to romanticize the beauty, the grace, the
"right" of a natural death. That when in the "Latest Decalogue,"
Arthur Hugh Clough tried with bitter sarcasm to chide us for our
indifference to the plight of the dying, his couplet should be
taken a century later as the slogan of the death with dignity
movement.*

The concept of "natural death" has crept up on us. We are not
sure what it means for death to be natural and yet are quite
certain it is a good thing. The concept has public policy implications — dangerous implications it seems to me. If death is not
only natural, but good somehow because it is natural, then as a
matter of public policy we ought not combat it. Perhaps the time
has come for a full blown exploration of the impact of this
seductively alluring concept. We may find that the temptress is
not without her dangers. Those who dance at Death's festival
may find that she has lured them with false promises; the morn-
ing after — if there be one — may be filled with lurid memories
of the night before.

---

*Of the fact that he was indeed poking fun at the philosophical gamesmanship
which distinguishes between killing and letting people die, there can be no
doubt from the other lines of his updating of God's message to Moses:
> Thou shall not steal; an empty feat
> when its so lucrative to cheat.
> Thou shalt not covet; but tradition
> aproves all forms of competition.

153

Dylan Thomas has become the straw man of the death with dignity movement when he urges us to "Rage, rage against the dying of the light." We poke fun at his pathological resistence to that which is clearly natural and inevitable. Certainly, in the case of the Welsh poet, the struggle was not terribly fruitful. He died at thirty-nine. Yet it may be that in this strange world where the artificial has become the natural, the heroic the expected, and the eternal punishment for Adam's sin a glory to be praised, a time has come to make a case for the goodness of life, even for the ideal of immortality.

In this paper I hope to make that case, or at least to make it *prima facie*. In the end I shall argue that the concept of natural death is at least dreadfully ambiguous and dangerous and possibly romantically elitist. If prolonging of physical life even to the point of immortality is an ideal long cherished by the common man and consistent with the most profound image of the human and the human community, we should prepare for profound policy dilemmas. That realistically the ideal will never be achieved and other policy goals are also crucial for that image of the human and the human community means that the case for immortality will in the end only be a modest one and that the task of complex research in economics and philosophy confronts us.

First I want to examine some of the public policy issues at stake by presenting two scenarios for the working out of the concept in public policy. Once some of the issues are presented it will be necessary to clarify some of the terms and make some basic analytical distinctions. Then I will give two arguments for supporting research designed to prevent certain deaths and ideally even death itself. Once the arguments have been made, I want to examine some of the cases for death and against immortality. Finally, I want to discuss why the case for ever extending life can only be a *prima facie* one, why two qualifications are necessary in a public policy designed to prolong healthy physical life without limit.

I. Natural Death: Its Public Policy Impact

At this point in history much more rides on the outcome of the debate that death is a good or an evil than it did in the day of

Socrates. When the traditional arguments have been made against the physical immortality of the body, little more has rested on the outcome than the mental satisfaction of an elite of Athens. Philosophers have always tried to resolve one of life's great philosophical dilemmas: Why it is that man must die?

Even if the struggle over the meaning of death once had a rather esoteric quality, as soon as death became a "natural" phenomenon it had political policy implications — or at least that is Ivan Illich's thesis.[1] He claims that from the first signs in the fifteenth century of the shift in man's understanding of death as a supernatural messenger from God to a natural force, the impact was to keep the doctor away from the death-bed of the peasant. By the eighteenth century humans had become unequal in death as in life. Death in active old age had become the ideal for elites. The leisure class could live longer because their lives had become less extenuating. They refused to retire because an expanding bureaucracy favored the ageless who had been around for a long time. By the nineteenth century, according to Illich, health had become a privilege of waiting for natural death. Industrial workers began demanding the right to medical and retirement insurance. Finally with the union movement, demands for equality in death produced a proletarian form of natural death. Workers were redefined as health care consumers, a move which first had revolutionary potential, but soon became a means of social control. Man now feels obliged to die a natural death. The right to die a natural death has become a duty. The physician now gives the patient "permission to die."[2] Biomedical intervention — a condition for a natural death — becomes compulsory, unless special dispensation is received.

It is clear that making complex biomedical technologies necessary for a natural death was a blatant contradiction which could not survive long. Nor could the radical egalitarianism of the proletarian form of natural death. It is natural that someone would seize upon the ambiguities in the term "natural," that a death with dignity movement would recognize that the artifacts of biomedical technology need not be called natural. Those who no longer need worry about the life's necessities — food, shelter, and especially medical care — now seem to have discovered the right to die the new natural death.

If that is the case, then Illich's clever analysis might be open to reinterpretation. He sees the proletariat enslaved by a medical elite demanding what the "health consumer" has been taught is the natural death of the intensive care unit. But it could also be that the elite is outflanking the masses, preparing the ground for a new stage in the combat — a stage where a basically healthy group can undermine the newly won right to life extending medical interventions. The new natural death is the new gnosis, accepted willingly by the enlightened and enforced upon the masses.

Whether Illich's interpretation and this reinterpretation of the modern history of natural death are correct, today the question of whether death is a good or an evil is argued for much higher stakes. Budgets of the National Institutes of Health depend upon whether conquering of arteriosclerosis in old age ought to get more or less priority than death in infancy from rare genetic disease. They depend on whether it is more important to extend the life span of those already living or to overcome the problems of infertility plaguing as much as ten percent of the married couples of the society. They depend upon whether natural death or natural weather disasters producing very unnatural deaths ought to get the greater share of the national resources.

An estimated $49,643,000,000 was spent in fiscal 1973 by the federal government alone on problems related to aging. Most of this was in support and social services for the elderly. Of that a comparatively tiny $12,300,000 was spent on medical research on the aging process, this by the National Institute of Child Health and Human Development. Excluded, however, are the $426 million for cancer research and $247 million for research on heart disease, the two diseases with public images of being enemies of natural death. The recent debates about the bill establishing the National Institute of Aging will provide a focus for research on the aging process and probably additional funding.

Drugs as diverse as procaine, vitamin E, and butylated hydroxytolvene (BHT), which may significantly extend the life span, are now in various stages of research and clinical trial in the United States.[3] A set of plausible theories accounting for a general aging process now focuses on genetic programming of the cell's DNA, protein and enzyme theories (such as synthetase function), the build up of free chemical radicals, surplus monoamine oxidase, cross-linkage formation, and autoimmune damage which may or may not be related to errors in cell replication.[4] Admittedly, extending the life span by twenty or forty years would not produce immortality, but it would extend life well beyond what is now thought "natural," and it would produce a radical social, political, and psychological change in society. If a natural death is a good to which all are entitled, then this research is malicious. If we still live after the fall when man is entitled to his three score years and ten and no more, then pharmacologists are trying to bite the fruit of the tree of life, the tree from which Adam and Eve were deprived when they were forced from the garden. Adam's most recent descendents have gained that knowledge of good and evil which is the fruit of that first fruit. Now they must decide whether Gerovital being tested in Nathan Kline's hospital ward for its life extending properties is an antidote for that apple or merely a synthetic and more flavorful modernization of that first temptation. The Food and Drug Administration, however, must make a choice. Unlike Plato's inquisitive colleagues in speculation, the FDA must have an answer. Should they decide that tasting this new fruit is as evil as was biting the first, then they must decide how they will regulate it under the present requirements of safety and effectiveness — the mandates of the FDA since the Kefauver amendment.

In order to present the policy implications of the concept of natural death most starkly, let me sketch two scenarios for the future of the concept over the next decade or two.

Natural Death: Two Scenarios

1. *The Dignified Death Scenario:*
    Death Ought to be Natural

The world of the dignified death is the world of Marya Mannes,[5] the signers of the Humanist's "Plea for Beneficent Euthanasia,"[6] and sometimes the Euthanasia Educational Council. Over the next decade fiefdoms for a dignified death will emerge. Walter Sackett will convince the representatives in the Florida State House to pass his legislation for death with dignity just as in the past year he has convinced his fellow Senators. Gradually other states will catch on. Oregon, West Virginia, Massachusetts, Idaho, Montana — all of whom have already considered legislation — will make clear that patients and patients' agents have the right to refuse medical treatments. The Living Will will be discussed in Protestant churches from Darien to Palo Alto. The recently developed Catholic Hospital Association version will spread among Catholics.

Since the Living Will is not a legally binding instrument (because it says it is not), Sidney Rosoff, legal counsel for the Euthanasia Educational Council and the American Civil Liberties Union, will be brought into a law suit. Eighty-seven year old Clarence Connolly will have signed a Living Will and lapsed into coma. His daughter, Hortence, serving as guardian, will ask to have the respirator turned off and will end up in court. Mrs. Martinez's case in Miami will be used as a precedent. Seventy-two year old Mrs. Martinez screamed her protests against continual cut downs on veins in her legs until she convinced her physician to go to court. Mrs. Martinez was ruled incompetent to make such a crucial judgment for herself so her daughter was appointed her agent. She affirmed her mother's refusal and Judge Popper let the guardian's refusal stand — the only case other than Karen Quinlan's of which I know where a court condoned a guardian's refusal of death prolonging medical treatments. But this was only a circuit court decision. Hortence Connolly will have to win her case on its merits.

Medical ethics courses will complement clinical instruction in medical schools so that physicians will gradually if reluctantly abandon what Francis Bacon called the third and new duty of the physician: the prolongation of life. The grounds will be that in medicine physicians have always believed that every case is so unique that no general rules can apply. Decisions will have to be made about continuing treatment on a case by case basis.

Meanwhile the country will still be in the latest stages of its third major depression. Pressures will surface for cutting the national budget — as a humane act of compassion to curb inflation. Since national defense cannot be compromised, sacrifices will have to be made in the domestic sphere. The National Institutes of Well-Being (NIW) and its parent Department of Health (formerly Health, Education and Welfare) will have to make a twenty percent budget cut.

At this point someone will realize that we are spending billions of dollars of the Department of Health's budget to prevent our distinguished senior citizens from exercising the well earned right to die with dignity. It is bizarre indeed for a government, which by then will have as its sole task the protection of the health of its citizens, to be engaged in such unhealthy behavior as combating nature's own way of giving meaning to life. Hortense Connolly and Judge Popper will have not simply a right, but a duty to promote a natural death.

2. *The Death is Evil Scenario:*
   No Death is Natural

Natural death may have a rather different future over the next decade or two. In this scenario we will discover that "natural death" is nothing more than a temporary accident in human history arriving in the fifteenth century as man begins to discard the accretions of supernaturalism and departing in about 1984 when we realize that no death is a natural death. In this scenario the pathologist is prophet. For him today as for the rest of us tomorrow, something always "causes" death. It never just happens. If the pathologist's view dominates, we may be at a transient moment in history where some deaths are thought caused by specific disease processes or acts of man, but others are just the natural wearing out of the machinery. At the present time, the non-pathologists among us still are able to think of deaths caused by specific diseases and voluntary acts of man as controllable, as potentially conquerable if we are aggressive enough in applying Western ingenuity and modern biomedical technologies. The goal is to let everyone spend his 80 or 90 years wandering the face of the earth so that death may come the way nature intended it.

Research on aging may change that. The work of Hayflick, Strehler, Goldstein, Comfort, and others begins to suggest that that "natural" limit may be subject to human control. In the

No-Death-Is-Natural future, every death will be seen as caused by humanly controlled events and potentially subject to human control. Deaths will be of three types, each someone's responsibility. One large group of deaths will be caused by the deceased's own behavior. Heart attacks are already thought caused in part by bad diet, poor exercise, smoking, and other controllable behaviors. The first critical development was really the germ theory of disease and the recognition that there were things we could do to keep microorganisms out of our bodies. Deaths resulting from failure to take medicines or have proper immunizations before foreign travel would now be thought to be a culpable death risking behavior. Cervical cancer in the woman who has failed to have a pap smear and automobile "accident" injury for one not wearing seat belts are now inevitably on their way to being voluntarily induced medical conditions.

Second, there will be those diseases that are the responsibility of one's parents. If Tay-Sachs disease is evil and predictable, can acceptance of the risk of the disease be anything other than voluntary and culpable behavior? Parental culpability is clearly a growth category.

Finally, there will be those deaths for which the NIW is responsible. To be convinced that a particular death is the result of potentially controllable processes and not make the societal effort to understand and control those processes is a voluntary political choice. It may well come to be seen as a culpable choice, especially if those afflicted are senile, or children, or otherwise incapable of making a rational claim that they are happy in their condition. In any case, the notion that there is no responsibility for getting a disease — a concept which has been the core of the medical model — will be short-lived. If no death is natural, death will be seen as even more evil than it is now; individual deaths will be seen as the responsibility of someone or some group.

— — —

While both scenarios are caricatures with unpalatable elements, I think a case can be made that the second view — that death is combatable and ought to be combatted — is the more human course. Much depends on the meaning of the term "natural" and upon some distinctions which must be made if we are to be clear in formulating a policy about death. It also depends on our conception of "the human."

II. Distinctions Needing To Be Made

A. The Meaning of the "natural"

"Natural death" is not the only place where the term natural is encountered in doing ethics and the life sciences. We have a frustratingly rich tradition of natural contraception, natural foods, natural drugs, natural sexual preferences, and natural instincts. Equally frustrating is the closely related concept of the "normal" as in normal behavior, normal intelligence, normal life span, and normal temperature. Standing behind some uses of both terms is an ethical/legal tradition of natural law.

The concept of the "natural" is one of the most used, misused, and abused in the field. It is central to both the fields of ethics and the life sciences. Before examining the policy implications of the concept of natural death, a brief linguistic analysis of the term 'natural' will be helpful. There are at least five distinct conceptions of the natural:

1. *The statistical.* The natural is the "usual," that which is the modal or near the mean. It is "natural" for a couple to prefer that their first child be a male. It is natural for man to die, in fact so natural that the class of those who do not may be a null class. Certainly it is limited to those humans who have been born in the past 100 or 150 years with possibly very few exceptions who are thought god-like for their unique properties. The opposite of natural in this sense is "unusual." It is clearly impossible to draw any policy conclusions about what we *ought* to do from this empirical description of the natural without an additional evaluative premise. To be ordinary is not necessarily to be right.

2. *The Biological.* The natural is that which occurs "among the animals" or "among the higher animals" or "according to man's biological nature." It is natural for humans to desire food and sexual activity, to avoid pain, and to die. Most if not all forms of contraception are unnatural in that the animal species do not practice them. Those who seek the normative from man's biological nature — an Epicurus, a Nietzsche, a Spencer, or a Darwin —

are very interested in this sense of the natural. It should be clear, though, that as with the statistical use of the term, another premise is needed to reach policy conclusions from this biological descriptive use of the term natural. The needed premise, that what occurs in animals is good or right, and good or right for man, seems most implausible.

3.   *The Anthropological.* The natural is that which occurs in nature, that which is not man-made or processed. Detergents are artificial; soap is natural. Dannon Yogurt is one hundred percent natural; it contains no artificial ingredients. It all comes straight from the cow without any man-made chemicals added. The opposite of natural in this sense is cultural, artificial, or artifactual. The distinction between the natural and the man-made seems to be a very primitive one. Levi-Strauss in *The Raw and the Cooked* analyzes myth systems for their symbolic differentiation of the world into the natural and the cultural.[7] Talcott Parsons distinguishes between those deaths which American society conceives to be natural and those caused by disease or accident which he calls "adventitious."[8] A death by murder or by automobile accident is not natural in the sense that it is caused by man's intervention into the natural. In the cult of the "back to nature movement" we affirm that if it is natural (not man-made) it is good. Once again the evaluative premise is needed. Stated in its most bold form — that all that is man-made is evil, and all that comes raw from the state of nature is good — it is certainly wrong. Some of man's interventions must be evil on balance. That is the judgment of those who are repulsed by the tubes and tracheostomy and technicians which keep the corpse respiring in the modern intensive care unit. But by this same notion disease caused by the "natural" invasion of the body by pathological microorganisms would have to be thought of as good, while the antibiotics (or at least synthetic ones) which save the child from his pneumonia, an evil. Artificiality, by itself, cannot be sufficient to declare an innovation an evil.

4.   *The Religious.* The natural is that which is part of the creation as opposed to the "supernatural," i.e., the events and forces which result from direct divine activity. There is a parallel dualism between the natural/supernatural dichotomy and the nature/artifact dichotomy. Levi-Strauss's Hegelian dualism is

also at home with the natural/supernatural distinction of the Greeks, Thomas, and Eastern conceptions of nature. Illich has claimed that the notion that death is a natural, rather than a supernatural, event is a uniquely modern phenomenon.

5. *The Moral.* The reason the natural and natural death cause us so much trouble at the policy level is that natural can also mean "moral." The natural is that which is in accord with the nature of man and the nature of the universe. Murdering innocent children is unnatural for man. Lying, war-making, hatred can be unnatural even if they are ubiquitous. Classical natural law tradition — Ulpian's trichotomous theory of law, the Stoics, Thomas, Troeltsch, and modern Catholic moral theologians — all understand the moral to be natural. So does the contemporary naturalist tradition in metaethics.[9]

The problem arises when the conception of the natural is applied in two or more senses simultaneously. This may happen in three ways: (1) A particular object or event may fit more than one conception, e.g., "It is natural (statistical and biological) for grass to be green." (2) It may also happen when certain schools of thought hold that one conception of the natural provides the content for another conception. "To determine what is natural (moral) for man, see what is in accord with his (biological) nature. This is Ulpian's *ius naturale* formulation. (3) Finally, the multiple conceptions of the natural may occur as fallacious arguments. "I have demonstrated that homosexuality is unnatural (statistical and maybe biological meanings). Therefore, since it is unnatural (moral meaning), it should not be practiced." "Death is a natural event (statistical, biological, non-supernatural); therefore, the scientifically trained expert should determine when natural (i.e., morally significant) life ceases." Making these leaps is what G.E. Moore called the naturalistic fallacy. Frankena persuasively refutes Moore's argument, though, by claiming that what really must be attacked is defining something into moral categories by demonstrating that it fits empirically into a certain nonmoral category *without defending the claim that such a definition is justified.*[10]

The problem with the concept of the natural death is that while death is clearly statistically natural and biologically natural, and presumably is natural in the sense of not being caused by divine spirits, it is not clear whether natural deaths are always to be preferred to man-made ones. Presumably all agree that adventitious deaths by gun shots or rampaging automobiles are not desirable, but there is utter chaos in deciding whether deaths prolonged by technological interventions are better or worse than those brought about by nature's uninterrupted course. The critical problem for public policy is whether such deaths are to be evaluated as good or as evil. Are they moral because they are natural or should they be conquered if possible through the use of man's rational capacity for technological intervention?

B.   Specific and Systemic Causes of Death

The received tradition gives us two types of antagonists to natural death: specific and systemic. Parsons, astute as he is in observing culture, seems to accept that adventitious deaths can be clearly distinguished from the category of "the inevitable 'natural' deaths of all individuals." [11] Specific causes of death are normally thought to interfere with natural death by making death premature. But the death with dignity movement has made us aware that the biomedical assault on these specific death causes can also make us view arteriosclerosis as natural and the struggle against it as artificial and evil. Thus specific diseases can interfere with natural death both by hastening it and by creating a situation where death is unnaturally prolonged. Even Parsons holds on to the notion that there is a natural, inevitable death which will occur if we only leave the body alone and give it a chance.

The field of gerontology is rapidly emerging as a new science with a rather old set of conceptual tools. Even the leaders in research on the aging process accept the view that the systemic aging process, "the biological clock," is fundamentally different from specific diseases. Leonard Hayflick speaks of the death of cells and the destruction of tissues and organs as a "normal part of morphogenic or developmental sequences." [12] Harman views the human as having a "natural human maximum life span." The basic aging processes have diseased states "superimposed and intertwined." [13]

This commonly received view may not stand scrutiny. The generalization often made that conquering specific diseases such as heart disease and cancer would add little to the life span appears to rest on the model of total system collapse after a "natural" life span. This in turn requires two assumptions. One, that other disease systems (respiratory and neurological) will not in turn be mastered leading to further life expectancy extensions and, two, that the aging process is not itself a "disease" or set of "diseases" subject to medical control. Most of the theories of aging, though, appear to lend themselves to medical intervention. Anti-oxidants may bind free radicals. Autoimmune reactions may be controlled with the emerging techniques of immunology. Genes programmed for aging may be controlled with genetic engineering. Monoamine oxidase inhibitors or appropriate analogues may correct enzyme defects. The view that aging is somehow different from disease may be wrong. The famous graphs showing life expectancy at birth approaching asymptotically to eighty-five years and capable of modification with age span or biological clock modifiers may simply be a product of a false dichotomy between natural life span and disease-induced shortening of that span. That arteriosclerosis and phenylketonuria are considered diseases but free radical accumulation or synthetase malfunction are considered "natural aging" may be a temporary accident of history. If distinguishing the natural and the abnormal has policy implications — as it apparently does in the minds of many — then clarifying such distinctions will be crucial for priorities in research and clinical health care.

C   *Socio-economic and Philosophical Problems of Immortality*

The fifty billion dollars spent yearly on aging, primarily for services to the elderly, makes clear the enormous social and economic problems in modifying the life span. Several authors have pointed out the phenomenal impact on our social institutions if we tamper with the aging process. If the years of retirement are significantly changed the social security system will require radical reorganization. The labor force, housing market, family structure, political alliances, and to some extent the population size will change. The calculation of just the economic impact of extending life expectancy by ten years would be an incredibly large task.

As critical and complex as these social and economic problems would be, there is a separate set of issues which really should be dealt with first. These are the philosophical-ethical problems of whether such life-extending innovations are good, independent of the social and economic costs. A strong case has been made in the history of philosophy for the goodness of death. If death's defenders are correct and influence policy accordingly, then the social and economic problems will be avoided. This paper concerns itself only with these latter problems — whether death is really an evil to be conquered in the first place.

D. Extended Mortal Life and Immortality

If it is concluded that life is indeed a good and death is an evil, then, two alternatives are conceivable: extended mortal life and immortality. It is possible to find either alternative good in theory while judging the other unacceptable. One might conclude, for instance, that immortality would be ideal, but that extended mortal life (which is all that we can realistically hope for) is no better than our present finite existence. If it all must end, then what does it matter when? On the other hand some might find the prospect of immortality unbearable, but the option of an additional 20-40 years quite attractive.

Since extended mortal life is a much more plausible outcome of human endeavor than immortality, the most difficult problem is presented by the individual who finds immortality an ideal utopia, but mere extension of mortal life of no value. The Stoics distinguished two natural laws: one, more absolute, was the law of the utopia; the other was the relative natural law for the real world. Pacifism might be an absolute law of nature, while a just war theory might be appropriate for the real and sinful world. I have always found one of the most perplexing dilemmas in philosophy to be whether one ought to pursue an ideal which he has reason to believe can never be achieved, or whether he ought to accommodate to the real world and pursue the relative ideal which is the best course once one concedes that the ideal cannot be achieved. Building the perfect jail is conceding that crimes will be committed. Establishing peer review committees is conceding that individual researchers will not always make the wisest, most detached judgments.

The idealist holds that one should not deviate from the telos; that approaching the real goal is better than achieving the substitute.[14] We in fact do not abandon the ideals of love, peace, and justice simply because we know they cannot be achieved, but realists do modify their behavior because they cannot not be perfectly achieved. The fact that the quest for immortality will only lead to extended mortal life would not dissuade the idealist even if he thinks that extended mortal life would be no gain. The realist, on the other hand, may have to be convinced that extended mortal life is a good in itself. This desire for extended mortal life appears to be in accord with the normal behavior of most humans and may be a sufficient justification for policy commitment to life extension even in the face of the reality of failure to achieve the eschaton. Commitment to life prolonging efforts, then, may have two independent justifications: the idealist's quest for immortality or the realist's desire for extended mortal life. At the policy level, it may not be necessary to distinguish the justifications if identical policies result.

III. The Cases For Life

It seems strange to make a case for life. Like happiness, truth, freedom, or justice, life seems to be an intrinsic good. Yet philosophers have been remarkably ingenious in putting forth arguments why the ending of life is not necessarily an evil. In fact I believe life is not an intrinsic good in the same way that happiness, truth, freedom or justice are. On the other hand, it is not simply an instrumental value either. If we are forced to make arguments against death and for life, presumably they must have more substance than the gut level affirmation of the pro-life movement. When pressed, two arguments seem cogent.

A. The Rationalist Case for Life

The first argument is that of the rationalist. Life should be affirmed as good and death as evil if it is consistent with promotion of the prudent, personal self-interest of the rational person. This argument is really history's response to Epicurus' frustratingly coherent argument that we should not fear death, that "so long as we exist death is not with us; but when death comes, then we do not exist."[15] Epicurus is convincing in dispelling fear of what comes after the moment of death — providing, of course, that when death comes I really do not exist. He does not, however, convince me that I should not fear the process of dying. More significantly, he does not convince me that I should not anticipate with regret the non-existence of my self. Since the fear of dying is uniquely horrifying because of the anticipatory regret of my non-existence, it is really the latter which leads me to the proposition that my death is an evil for me.

But why this anticipatory regret? There are many future states which I desire. Some have nothing to do with me; they will occur or fail to occur quite independent of my existence. Others involve me in some way or another. Some of those involving me I desire only on the condition that I am alive. An example is my desire to have my pension.[16] The desired future state in that case in no way makes me desire to continue to live. A second group of future states I desire involve me because I think I am able to promote those states better if I am alive. My desire that my children receive a college education is an example. Finally, some of the future states I desire involve me because I must be present. My desire to complete my research on my favorite project or my desire to see my children graduate from college require that I be around. These desires differ from my pension in that for the pension I desire that it exist only if I am around, but for the research and the commencement I desire to be around in order to have those experiences. For anyone who has desires about future states requiring his own existence, it is rational that he regret the anticipation of his non-existence.

That I may desire my existence, of course, does not demonstrate that it is desirable that I continue to exist, much less that the state has a reason to undertake efforts to see that I continue to exist. The fact that many people have in common the desire for future states which require their existence does, however, create a common interest. To the degree, however, that the state has a legitimate interest in promoting the general welfare, and particularly promoting it when the individual efforts of individual citizens taken separately would not be effective, the state may prudently adopt a policy of conducting research and providing medical services which will tend to promote that general welfare. Prudent individuals form a contract to achieve together what they cannot achieve separately.

While this may provide an argument that the state can legitimately support death-averting programs, I do not think it is the strongest argument. First, it may confuse the desired and the desirable. That I desire future states requiring my existence does not make my future existence a good and my death an evil. That the vast majority of citizens desire their future existence does not mean promotion of their future existence by the state right. Second, and I believe more devastating, the case for life and against death based on the prudence of the rational individual contracting with other individuals is, in the end, both too egocentric and too individualistic. A stronger argument for life and against death, I believe, rests in what, for lack of a better label, I will call the social-eschatological case.

B. The Social-Eschatological Case for Life

To argue the evilness of death is to argue man's place in the cosmos. Man must come to grips with death in terms of his understanding of his nature and his vision of his place in the telos — the ideal world toward which we strive. Western man is incessantly teleological. He dreams of a Kingdom of God which is a social, political reality — Kingdom is a very political metaphor. He dreams of life immortal (if he is influenced by the Greeks) or of resurrection of the body (if one prefers the Christian vision). In the combining of the two strands of our heritage, the body has won a place for itself from which we need never again feel we must escape. Common to all the significant Western eschatologies is a vision of perpetuation. While the pre-Christian Jewish tradition devoted relatively little attention to the problem of death, it transmitted the belief that death is the wages of sin. At least by the period of the Maccabees, it also had a vision of a Messiah who would atone for that sin and create a perpetual Kingdom.

Modern Western man is deeply rooted in this social eschatology. Anticipated in the Johannine realized eschatology, it becomes much more this worldly in the modern era. Man prays, "Thy Kingdom come on earth," and means it. He is an activist who sees it as part of his task to bring into reality that vision of the new world, the world where evil is no more. And one of the evils which he has dreamed about conquering is the evil of death. His social vision is one which he himself must play a part in constructing — and one in which life can be prolonged through the use of man's ingenuity to master diseases one by one. Life shall be a struggle. But in the end the goodness of life is to be affirmed. Man shall have dominion over the earth and subdue it. Life shall prevail and death shall be no more.

If this social eschatology is the basis for a commitment to a governmental policy of prolongation of life, we need not be confined to the individualism of the rationalist. Overcoming of death — my own and my fellow man's — is the final step in the overcoming of evil and the building of human community.

> Any man's death diminishes me, because I am involved in Mankind; And therefore never send to know for whom the bell tolls; It tolls for thee.

IV. The Cases For Death and Against Immortality

Against this vision stands a long line of argument from Plato and Aristotle through Darwin to Hartshorne, Morison and Kass. Five arguments I have identified as potent counters thrust against the goals of extended mortal life or the ideal of immortality. Each shall be examined in turn.

A. Death as Relief from Suffering

Perhaps the most common case to be made for death is that it is the great liberator. The poet cloys with death's sweetness:

> Come lovely and soothing death,
> Undulate round the world, serenely, arriving, arriving,
> In the day, in the night, to all, to each

Sooner or later, delicate death.
Prais'd be the fathomless universe,
For life and joy, and for objects and knowledge curious,
And for love, sweet love — But praise! praise! praise!
For the sure-enwinding arms of cool-enfolding death.[17]

That death can be the great liberator was clear to Socrates. Plato
has Socrates say in the *Crito*, "When man has reached my age, he
ought not to be repining at the approach of death." While in
Plato's account escaping the miseries of old age plays a secondary role for Socrates, in Xenophon it becomes the main reason
for Socrates' uncompromising position before his judges.

Do you know that I would refuse to concede that any man has
lived a better life than I have up to now? . . . But now, if my years
are prolonged, I know that the frailties of old age will inevitably
be realized. . . . Perhaps God in his kindness is taking my part and
securing me the opportunity of ending my life not only in season
but also in the way that is easiest.[18]

In speaking of ending his life "in season" Socrates is the
original advocate of the naturalness of death. Xenophon has
Socrates say, "Have you not known all along from the moment of
my birth nature has condemned me to death." But now, that
condemnation by nature to a natural death is being challenged.
The choice need not be as with Socrates between "the frailties of
old age" and death, but between death and medical treatments
which potentially will prolong the prime of life and conquer at
least some of the debilitating diseases from which death was the
humane release.

B. Death as Relief from Boredom

A related case for death and against immortality is made by
those who fear the unbearable tedium of an endless life. To be
condemned to eternal life is a Sartre-esque torture of enormous
proportion. Here the distinction between extended mortal life
and immortality may be crucial. Those who believe they fear
immortality more than death may be quite delighted with a few
score more years for completion of their earthly projects. The
case for death as a relief from the boredom of immortality does
not create a problem for those who advocate a public policy of

support for research to extend the life span based on the basis of the good of extended mortal life. If, however, immortality would be boring, it does present a formidable challenge to the other principle upon which support for such research is based, the principle that ever-extending life is the ideal toward which we strive.

Does this argument against the ideal work? I think not. I find in it a hollow, sour-grapes quality which might be satisfying to some philosophers, but would be rather unconvincing to a broader public. Bernard Williams has articulated the argument based on the play by Karel Capek in which a woman named Elina Makropulos was given an elixar of life by her father, a sixteenth-century Emperor. At the time of the play she is 342 and lives, apparently physically healthy, but in a state of boredom, indifference, and coldness.[19]

It is Williams' argument, as I understand it, that it is not an accident of her particular life that she is bored, but that it is essential to human nature that an endless life would be a meaningless one.[20] Elina Makropulos's problem, according to Williams, is that "everything that could happen and make sense to one particular human being . . . had already happened."[21] He then maintains that the fact that life ceased to have meaning for her, that she "frose up," is essential to human nature and not dependent on her particular contingent character or the fact that others around her did not share her immortal capacities.

In developing his arguments he considers several alternatives: one continuous life, a series of lives connected by a common memory, and theories of an after-life. The core of the argument, though, focuses on the primary case of one continuous life. Williams argues that two conditions would have to be met for the prospect of living forever to be attractive: (1) that it should clearly be *me* who lives forever and (2) "that the state in which I survive should be one which, to me looking forward, will be adequately related, in the life it presents, to those aims which I now have in wanting to survive at all."[22]

I readily concede the first condition. It poses no problem for the kind of ideal relevant to public policy for research on aging. It *would* be me who lives forever. The second condition is more difficult. It includes two component arguments: (1) that it is irrational to pursue a future desire if it is clearly impossible to achieve it and (2) that it is impossible to have an infinite agenda of categorical desires (desires requiring my presence for their fulfillment).

Williams does not explicitly deal with either of these claims. I think both can be challenged. The first, that it is irrational to hold as an ideal, a state which we recognize cannot be achieved, we have already discussed. I find the position implausible, especially when *holding* that ideal would reasonably lead us *toward* that ideal even though it cannot realistically be achieved and when approaches to the ideal are considered progressively better in and of themselves. The second, forces us to deal with the claim that it is essential to human nature that boredom will eventually be the result of living forever, that Elina Makropulos's plight was not an accident of her personality, but essential to the human condition.

This position requires the presumption that man necessarily has finite categorical desires or that he at least has a finite capacity to develop new ways of fulfilling all of those desires. If my more eschatological understanding of man as a community builder is correct, I see no reason why this must be the case. If man's hopes are infinite, it is possible to continually have hope of fulfilling some categorial desires while at the same time not fulfilling all of them. If the vision is utopian, the possibility of new and fulfilling experiences is infinite. Furthermore some realistic categorical desires, some of the most important ones, do not depend on the newness of experiences. The desire to live in a loving and happy relationship with one's family does not necessarily require continual novelty for its fulfillment. In fact such a relationship conceivably might be quite stable without inevitably leading to boredom. While the knowledge of death might enrich some such experiences by giving them a timely quality, it certainly also introduces great tragedy.

Finally, Williams appears to argue that for immortality to be attractive boredom must be unthinkable.[23] It could be that he is simply not a gambler and is not willing to take a chance unless he is assured of the success of an unboring immortality. If the ideal, however, of continual non-boring existence is really an ideal, it should not be necessary to rule out failure as "unthinkable" in order for one to be willing to give it a try. It might not be worth the gamble if the boring immortality were compulsory. Elina Makropulos's was not, however. She stopped taking the elixar and died. Certainly any realistic public policy efforts to combat death hold out the same escape. Compulsory immortality is not among the conceivable treatments. As long as continual fulfillment of categorial desires is possible, it would seem both that there is hope that total boredom might be avoided and that it was worth the risk — especially since failures can be aborted. On the contrary it would seem that the burden of proof would be on those who would hold that boredom is inevitable. I do not see that as either plausible or provable.

C. Death as a Source of Meaning

Teleologists may make their case for as well as against death. Death, it may be argued, gives life a sense of timeliness and purpose. This is the argument explored by Paul Ramsey, that death gives us reason to "number our days."[24] Were we to believe that we had forever to complete our projects, the sense of urgency and excitement in life would be lost. This is probably one of the most convincing cases for death faced by Judeo-Christian man, by man who is temporally oriented. Were immortality to come at the price of giving up a sense of time and timeliness, the price would be high indeed. But would that in fact be the result? Certainly not unless the eschatological ideal is achieved, but even then it is not clear why perpetual life would be a timeless life. The test of this objection to immortality, as with the previous one, rests with the man — the wise and the many. Would indeed humans who are not part of Illich's elite seriously consider abandoning the possibility of extending physical life in order to guarantee protection against endless boredom and loss of a sense of time? I think not.

D. Death as a Force for Progress

For this particularly modern argument for death we cite the poet Morison:

Every human death is ultimately for the good of the group. . . . To rage against death is to rage at the very process which made one a human in the first place.[25]

That evolution has depended upon the death of the weak so that the more fit may thrive is the first law of Darwin. To this point in history, it seems irrefutable. But need the evolutionist's position remain valid? To be sure, were immortality to be achieved, reproduction would have to cease — if population were to remain stable. But if mortal life is extended, the reproductive process would at the most merely be slowed. Even if biological evolution ceased completely, it is not clear to this author that at this point in history this would necessarily be an evil. For one who believes as firmly in progress as I, that may be heresy, but it is not at all clear to me that, for instance, continual evolution in intelligence so that more and more people have the intellectual capacities to build world-destroying weapon systems is an adaptive development. If evolution was once only biological, it may now be cultural as well. If continued adaptation is necessary for survival in an ever changing universe, possibly cultural adaption may be sufficient or even preferable.

E. *Natural Death as a Comforting Fiction*

We are left with one last ditch line of defense by the advocates of death. Natural death, they may concede, is nothing more than a fiction. Indeed deaths all do have a cause and that cause is potentially susceptible to research and control. But the fiction is a comforting one. It is agonizing to realize that every death, and the suffering which accompanies it, is the result of some human choice. Some human individual or group is responsible. Perpetuating the fiction of natural death at least relieves the common man of the burden of responsibility.

Relieve him it does, but at the expense of continuing the suffering of death striking out in random and unregulated viciousness. It is the death of the animal species, but in being so it is sub-human. If our vision of man is correct, if man is a responsible agent charged with the task of creating and sustaining his life and his environment, then such fictions are escapist. Freedom such fictions may give, but the result is a tyranny of freedom. To escape from responsibility to the comforts of natural death cannot be a sustainable defense.

V. Qualifications on A Public Policy of Prolonging Life

If prolonging of life and combatting of "natural" death are goods which are part of man's responsibility in the building of human community, problems still remain, problems hinted at in the arguments in favor of death. Socrates' choice of death over the frailties of old age anticipates the first.

A. Death as a Relative Rather than an Absolute Evil

To maintain that death is fundamentally incompatible with the ideal human community is not to say that death must always be fought. It is possible to maintain that immortality is a desirable goal and still hold that some deaths may be preferred to a painful and dehumanizing struggle to that goal. If death is an evil there still may be lives which are worse evils. Both the evil of death and the acceptability of individual deaths may be affirmed. To hold death as an evil and still feel that individual deaths are acceptable may be a tragic view of death; it may mean that "accidental" deaths and deaths from the culpable choices of individuals or governments may be seen as much more traumatic. The ideal, however, is not incompatible with Living Wills, legal documents to facilitate refusal of intolerable death prolonging medical treatments, and even legislation to clarify the right of individuals and their guardians to make such refusals. As an active participant in the movement for the right of the dying to refuse treatment, I write this present paper really as a footnote to correct any mistaken implication that affirming the evil of death and the relative acceptability of particular deaths is incompatible. Until the day of the eschaton, such tragic choices will still have to be made.

B. The Priorities Problem

If (and only if) life is worth prolonging and death is worth combatting, then the social and economic problems of policy choices become central. To make a case for immortality or extended mortal life is not to say conquering death has the highest of priorities on the human agenda. This is an allocation of resources question. The answer will depend upon both economic and social data and upon philosphical/ethical choices. If the total amount of good to come in a life is roughly proportional to the quality of life yet to be lived and if one opts for the utilitarian distributional principle of maximizing the total good, then research on aging and on overcoming causes of death late in life will receive very low priority. Even if the quantity of life can be extended without lowering the quality, research on diseases of infants and children surely will take priority. If, however, the good of a life is unrelated to quantity yet to be lived and/or the distributional principle is not the utilitarian one, then the priorities may be very different. If, for instance, the distributional principle is that medical resources should go first to those least well off — a plausible general principle of justice in health care delivery we shall support in a sequel to this paper — then the aging may have a much stronger claim to our health care dollars. If the aging constitute a minority group of the medically (and socially) disadvantaged, then perhaps a case can be made that justice demands special funding priority for their special concerns. That all of us who are fortunate will one day count ourselves among the aged can only make the policy determination more complex. To say that extending life is not of highest priority is radically different from saying that "natural" death is a good, a right, or a duty. It may be that we will conclude that giving everyone a reasonable chance to have a relatively normal life span free from pain and suffering is of higher priority than extending life. If so, let the implications fall where they may — let the dollars flow from the Cancer and Heart Institutes to those more oriented to pediatrics. But we should not in the process imply that our task will be complete if ever that goal should be achieved. If indeed life is a good, then short of achieving immortality, the struggle will continue. To hold otherwise is to concede that there are things we could do to extend life with high quality which we choose not to do. Our care of the elderly and dying demands more.

It was Euripides who said, "When death approaches old age is no burden." Modern man's revision might appropriately be "The less one has to fear that death is approaching, the less will be the burden of old age."

NOTES

1. Ivan Illich. "The Political Uses of Natural Death," *Hastings Center Studies* 2 (1974): 3-20.

2. Eric J. Cassell "Permission to Die," *Bioscience* 23 (1973): 475-78.

3. D. Harman, "Free Radical Theory of Aging," *Triangle* 12 (1973): 155; Harold M. Schmeck, "Disputed Drug Is Restudied for Use in Geriatrics," *The New York Times*, March 18, 1973, p. 57.

4. See Leonard Hayflick, "The Biology of Human Aging," *The American Journal of the Medical Sciences* 265 (1973): 432-445; A. Comfort, "Biological Theories of Aging," *Human Development* 13 (1970): 127-39; and Samuel Goldstein, "The Biology of Aging." *The New England Journal of Medicine* 285 (1971): 1120-1129.

5. Marya Mannes, *Last Rights: A Plea for the Good Death* (New York: William Morrow, 1974).

6. "A Plea for Beneficent Euthanasia," *The Humanist*, July/August, 1974, pp. 4-5.

7. Levi-Strauss, *The Raw and the Cooked* (New York: Harper, 1969).

8. Talcott Parsons and Victor Lidz, "Death in American Society," in *Essays in Self-Destruction*, ed. Edwin S. Shneidman (New York: Science House, 1967).

9. G. E. Moore, *Principia Ethica* (Cambridge, England: Cambridge University Press, 1903); W. K. Frankena, "The Naturalistic Fallacy," in *Readings in Ethical Theory,* ed. John Hospers and Wilfrid Sellars (New York: Appleton-Century-Crofts, Inc., 1952), pp. 103-114; Roderick Firth, "Ethical Absolutism and the Ideal Observer," *Philosophy and Phenomenological Research* 12 (1952): 317-345; Robert M. Veatch, "Does Ethics Have an Empirical Basis?" *Hastings Center Studies* 1 (1973): 50-65.

10. Frankena, "The Naturalistic Fallacy."

11. Parsons and Lidz, "Death in American Society."

12. Hayflick, "Biology of Human Aging," p. 442.

13. Harman, "Free Radical Theory of Aging," p. 154.

14. I am, of course, using the terms "idealist" and "realist" not in their technical philosophical meanings, but rather to contrast one who is guided by ideals and one who is influenced by more practical considerations.

15. Epicurus, "Epicurus to Monoeceus," in *Ethical Theories* ed. A.I. Melden (Englewood Cliffs, N.J.: Prentice-Hall, Inc., 1967), p. 144.

16. I am indebted to Bernard Williams for much of the argument presented in this paragraph. See his essay "The Makropulos Case: Reflections on the Tedium of Immortality," in *Problems of the Self* (Cambridge: University Press, 1973), pp. 82-100.

17. Walt Whitman. "When Lilacs Last in the Dooryard Bloom'd," *Leaves of Grass*.

18. See Jacques Choron, *Death and Western Thought* (New York: Collier Books 1963), p. 43.

19. See Williams, "The Makropulos Case."
20. *Ibid.*, p. 89.
21. *Ibid.*, p. 90.
22. *Ibid.*, p. 91.
23. *Ibid.*, p. 95.
24. Paul Ramsey, "The Indignity of 'Death with Dignity,' " *Hastings Center Studies* 2 (1974), 47-62.
25. Robert S. Morison, "The Last Poem: The Dignity of the Inevitable and Necessary," *Hastings Center Studies* 2 (1974), p. 66.

SELECTED BIBLIOGRAPHY

Agate, John. "Care of the Dying in Geriatric Departments." *Lancet* (February 17, 1973): 364-66.

Agich, George J. "The Concepts of Death and Embodiment," *Lancet*, February 17, 1973, 364-66.

Ariès, Philippe. *Western Attitudes toward Death: From the Middle Ages to the Present.* Trans. by Patricia M. Ranum. Baltimore: Johns Hopkins University Press, 1974.

Ayd, F. J., Jr. "The Hopeless Case: Medical and Moral Considerations." *Journal of the American Medical Association* 181 (1962): 1099-1102.

Bard, B. and Fletcher, J. "The Right to Die," *Atlantic* (April, 1968): 59-64.

Barton, David. "Death and Dying: A Psychiatrist's Perspective." *Soundings* 55 (Winter, 1972): 459-71.

Baughman, William H. "Euthanasia: Criminal Tort, Constitutional and Legislative Questions." *Notre Dame Lawyer* 48 (1973): 1202-60.

Bayles, Michael D. "Criminal Paternalism." In *The Limits of Law: Nomos XV,* ed. J. Roland Pennock and John W. Chapman. New York: Lieber-Atherton, 1974.

Becker, Ernest. *The Denial of Death.* New York: Free Press, 1973.

Beecher, Henry K. "After the 'Definition of Irreversible Coma'." *New England Journal of Medicine* 281 (November 6, 1960): 1070-71.

_____. "Ethical Problems Created by the Hopelessly Unconscious Patient." *New England Journal of Medicine* 278 (1968): 1425-30.

_____. "Procedures for the Appropriate Management of Patients Who May Have Supportive Measures Withdrawn." *Journal of the American Medical Association* 209 (1969): 405.

Black, Peter McL. "Three Definitions of Death," *The Monist* 60 (1977): 136-46.

Bok, Sisela, *et al.* "The Dilemmas of Euthanasia," *BioScience* 23 (August, 1973): 461-68.

Brierley, J. B., *et al.* "Neocortical Death after Cardiac Arrest," *The Lancet,* September 11, 1971, 560-65.

Brim, Jr., Orville G., *et al.,* eds. *The Dying Patient.* New York: Russell Sage Foundation, 1970.

Brody, Howard. "The Physician-Patient Contract: Legal and Ethical Aspects," *The Journal of Legal Medicine,* July/August 1976, 25-30.

Brown, Norman, *et al.* "The Preservation of Life." *Journal of the American Medical Association* 221 (January 5, 1970): 76-82.

Bulger, Roger J., ed. *Hippocrates Revisited.* New York: Medcom Press, 1973.

Burns, Chester R. and Engelhardt, Jr., H. T., eds. "The Humanities and

Medicine." *Texas Reports on Biology and Medicine.* Vol. 32, No. 1 (Spring, 1974).

Callahan, Daniel. "On Defining a 'Natural Death'," *The Hastings Center Report* 7 (June, 1977): 32-37.

Cantor, Norman L. "A Patient's Decision to Decline Life-Saving Medical Treatment: Bodily Integrity versus the Preservation of Life," *Rutgers Law Review* 26 (Winter, 1972): 228-64.

Capron, Alexander and Leon R. Kass. "A Statutory Definition of the Standards for Determining Human Death: An Appraisal and a Proposal." *University of Pennsylvania Law Review* 121 (1972): 87-118.

Cartwright, Ann, et al. *Life Before Death.* London: Routledge and Kegan Paul, 1973.

Casey, John, ed. *Morality and Moral Reasoning.* London: Methuen, 1971.

Cassell, Eric J. "Death and the Physician." *Commentary,* June, 1969, 73-79.

_____. "Permission to Die." *BioScience* 23 (August, 1973): 475-78.

_____. "Treating the Dying — The Doctor vs. The Man Within the Doctor," *Medical Dimensions,* 1 (1972), 6-11, 22.

_____. *The Healer's Art: A New Approach to the Doctor-Patient Relationship.* Philadelphia: J.B. Lippincott Company, 1976.

Caughill, Rita E., ed. *The Dying Patient: A Supportive Approach.* Boston: Little, Brown, 1976.

Choron, Jacques. *Death and Modern Man.* New York: Collier Books, 1964.

_____. *Death and Western Thought.* New York: Collier Books, 1973.

Collins, V. J. "Limits of Medical Responsibility in Prolonging Life: Guides to Decisions." *Journal of the American Medical Association* 206 (1968): 389-92.

Craven, Joan, and Wald, Florence S. "Hospice Care for Dying Patients," *American Journal of Nursing,* 75 (October, 1975): 1816-22.

"Diagnosis of Brain Death," *The Lancet,* November 13, 1976, 1069-70.

Dinello, Daniel. "On Killing and Letting Die," *Analysis 31* (January, 1971), 83-86.

Downie, P.A. "Symposium: Care of the Dying; A Personal Commentary on the Care of the Dying on the North American Continent," *Nursing Mirror,* 139 (October 10, 1974): 68-70.

Downing, A. B. *Euthanasia and the Right to Die.* New York: Humanities Press, 1970.

Duff, Raymond S. and A. G. M. Campbell. "Moral and Ethical Dilemmas in the Special-Care Nursery." *New England Journal of Medicine* 289 (October 25, 1973): 890-94.

Dworkin, Gerald. "Paternalism." In *Morality and the Law,* ed. Richard

A. Wasserstrom. Belmont, California: Wadsworth Publishing Company, Inc., 1971.

Dworkin, Roger B. "Death in Context," and Capron, Alexander M. "The Purpose of Death: A Reply to Professor Dworkin." *Indiana Law Journal* 48 (Summer, 1973): 623-48.

Elkinton, J. Russell. "The Dying Patient, The Doctor, and The Law." *Villanova Law Review* 13 (Summer, 1968): 740-750.

Engelhardt, H. Tristram, Jr. "The Counsels of Finitude," *Hastings Center Report* 5 (April 1975): 29-36.

Feifel, Herman, ed. *The Meaning of Death*. McGraw-Hill, 1959.

Feinberg, Joel. "Legal Paternalism." *Canadian Journal of Philosophy* 1 (1971): 105-24.

Flanagan, Dennis, ed. *Life and Death and Medicine*. San Francisco: W. H. Freeman & Co., 1973.

Fletcher, Joseph. *Morals and Medicine*. Boston: Beacon Press, 1954.

Foot, Philippa. "Euthanasia," *Philosophy and Public Affairs* 6 (1977): 85-112.

Freirich, Emil J. "The Best Medical Care for the 'Hopeless' Patient." *Medical Opinion*, February, 1972, 51-55.

Friends, Society of, *Who Shall Live? Man's Control over Birth and Death*. New York: Hill and Wang, 1970.

Garland, Michael. "The Right to Die in California — Politics, Legislation, and Natural Death," *Hastings Center Report* 6 (October, 1976): 5-6.

Garner, J. "Palliative Care: It's the Quality of Life Remaining That Matters," *Canadian Medical Association Journal* 115 (July 17, 1976): 179-80.

Gert, Bernard, and Charles M. Culver. "The Definition of Paternalism," *Philosophy & Public Affairs* 6 (1976): 45-57.

Goldberg, Ivan K., et al., eds. *Phychopharmacolgic Agents for the Terminally Ill and Bereaved*. New York: Columbia University Press, 1973.

Hancock, Sheila, et al. "Care of the Dying." *British Medical Journal*, January 6, 1973, 29-41.

Harvard Medical School, Ad Hoc Committee of the Harvard Medical School to Examine the Definition of Brain Death. "A Definition of Irreversible Coma." *Journal of the American Medical Association* 205 (1968): 337-40.

Heifetz, Milton D., with Charles Mangel. *The Right to Die: A Neurosurgeon Speaks with Candor*. New York: G.P. Putnam's Sons, 1975.

Hendin, David. *Death as a Fact of Life*. New York: Norton, 1973.

High, Dallas M. "Death: Its Conceptual Elusiveness." *Soundings* 55 (Winter, 1972): 438-58.

Hinton, J. M. *Dying*. Baltimore: Penguin Books, 1967.

Holden, Constance. "Hospices For the Dying, Relief from Pain and Fear," *Science* 30 (July, 1976).

Illich, Ivan. "The Political Uses of Natural Death," *Hastings Center Studies* 2 (January, 1974): 3-20.

Institute of Society, Ethics and the Life Sciences, Task Force on Death and Dying. "Refinements in Criteria for the Determination of Death." *Journal of the American Medical Association* 221 (July 3, 1972): 48-53.

In the Matter of Karen Quinlan: The Complete Legal Briefs, Court Proceedings, and Decision in the Superior Court of New Jersey, Arlington, Va.: University Publications of America. Vol. I, 1975; Vol. II, 1976.

Janzen, E. "Relief of Pain: Prerequisites to the Care and Comfort of the Dying," *Nursing Forum* 13 (1974): 48-51.

Johnson, Alan G. "The Right to Live or the Right to Die," *Nursing Times,* May 13, 1971, 575-577.

Jonas, Hans. "Against the Stream," *Philosophical Essays.* Englewood Cliffs, New Jersey: Prentice-Hall, 1974.

_____. *The Phenomenon of Life.* New York: Dell Publishing Co., 1966.

Kass, Leon. "Death as an Event: A Commentary on Robert Morison." *Science* 173 (August 20, 1971): 698-702.

Kennedy, Ian McColl. "The Kansas Statute on Death — An Appraisal." *New England Journal of Medicine* 285 (1971): 946-50.

Koenig, Ronald. "Dying vs. Well-Being," *Omega* 4 (Fall, 1973): 181-94.

Kohl, Marvin, ed. *Beneficent Euthanasia.* Buffalo: Prometheus Books, 1975.

_____. *The Morality of Killing.* New York: Humanities Press, 1974.

Krant, Melvin. *Dying and Dignity: The Meaning and Control of a Personal Death.* Springfield, Ill.: Charles C. Thomas, 1974.

Kübler-Ross, Elisabeth. *On Death and Dying.* New York: Macmillan, 1969.

_____. *Questions and Answers on Death and Dying.* New York: Macmillan & Co., 1974.

Lamerton, Richard. *Care of the Dying.* London: Priory Press Limited, 1973.

Mack, Arien, ed. *Death in the American Experience.* New York: Schocken, 1973.

Maguire, Daniel C. *Death By Choice.* New York: Doubleday, 1973.

Malone, Robert J. "Is There a Right to a Natural Death?" *New England Law Review* 9 (Winter 1974): 293-310.

May, William F. "Code, Covenant, Contract, or Philanthrophy," *Hastings Center Report* 5 (December, 1975): 29-38.

McCormick, S. J., Richard A. "To Save or Let Die: The Dilemma of

184 *Medical Treatment of the Dying*

Modern Medicine." *Journal of the American Medical Association* 229 (1974): 172-76.

McKinlay, John. "Who is Really Ignorant — Physician or Patient?" *Journal of Health and Social Behavior* 16 (March 1975): 3-11.

McNulty, B. J. "St. Christopher's Outpatients," *American Journal of Nursing* 71 (December, 1971): 2328-30.

_____. McNulty, B. J. "Discharge of the Terminally-ill Patient." *Nursing Times*, September, 1970: 1160-62.

Middleton, Carl L., Jr. "Principles of Life-Death Decision Making," *Linacre Quarterly* 42 (November 1975): 268-78.

Montange, Charles H. "Informed Consent and the Dying Patient." *Yale Law Journal* 83 (1974): 1632-64.

Morgan, Lucy Griscom. "On Drinking the Hemlock." *Hastings Center Report* 1 (December, 1971): 4-5.

Morison, Robert S. "Dying." *Scientific American* 229 (September, 1973): 55-62.

_____. "Death — Process or Event?" *Science* 173 (August 20, 1971): 694-98.

Neale, Robert E. "Between the Nipple and the Everlasting Arms." *Archives of the Foundation of Thanatology* 3 (Spring, 1971): 21-30.

_____. *The Art of Dying.* New York: Harper & Row, 1973.

"Optimum Care for Hopelessly Ill Patients. A Report of the Clinical Care Committee of the Massachusetts General Hospital," *New England Journal of Medicine* 295 (August 12, 1976): 362-64.

Parsons, Talcott, Renée C. Fox, and Victor M. Lidz. "The 'Gift of Life' and Its Reciprocation," *Social Research* 39 (1972): 367-415.

Pearson, Leonard, ed. *Death and Dying: Current Issues in the Treatment of the Dying Person.* Cleveland: Case Western Reserve U.P., 1969.

Perlin, Michael L. "The Right to Refuse Treatment in New Jersey," *Psychiatric Annals* 6 (June 1976): 90 ff.

Pius XII. "The Pope Speaks, Prolongation of Life." *Osservatore Romano* 4 (1957): 393-98.

Platt, Michael. "Commentary: On Asking to Die," *Hastings Center Report* 5 (Decemer 1975): 9-12.

Poteat, W. H. "I Will Die: An Analysis." *Philosophical Quarterly*, 9 (January 1959): 3-15.

Rabkin, Mitchell T., et al. "Orders Not to Resuscitate," *New England Jounal of Medicine* 295 (1976): 364-69.

Ramsey, Paul. *The Patient as Person.* New Haven: Yale University Press, 1970.

Robertson, John A. "Involuntary Euthanasia of Defective Newborns: A Legal Analysis." *Stanford Law Review* 27 (1975): 213-70.

Robitscher, Jonas. "The Right to Die." *Hastings Center Report* 2 (September, 1972): 11-14.

Russell, O. Ruth. *Freedom to Die: Moral and Legal Aspects of Euthanasia.* New York: Human Sciences Press, 1975 (New York: Dell Publishing Co., 1976).

Sackett, Walter W. "Death with Dignity," *Medical Opinion and Review* 5 (June, 1969): 25-31.

St. John Stevas, Norman. *The Right to Life.* New York: Rinehart and Winston, 1963.

Saunders, Cicely. *Care of the Dying.* London: Macmillan & Co., 1960.

_____. "The Last Stages of Life." *American Journal of Nursing* 65, (March, 1965): 70-75.

_____. "Living with Dying," with commentaries by Samuel C. Klagsbrun, Austin H. Kutscher, and Wayne Proudfoot. *Man and Medicine* 1 (Spring, 1976): 227-51.

Schulz, Richard, and David Aderman. "How the Medical Staff Copes with Dying Patients: A Critical Review," *Omega* 7 (1976): 11-21.

Scott, Charles E. "Reflections on Dying." *Soundings* 55 (Winter, 1972): 472-79.

Shils, E., et al. *Life or Death: Ethics and Options.* Seattle: University of Washington Press, 1968.

Smith, David H. "On Letting Some Babies Die." *Hastings Center Studies* 2 (May, 1974): 37-46.

Sollitto, Sharmon, and Robert M. Veatch. *Bibliography of Society, Ethics and The Life Sciences.* New York: A Hastings Center Publication, 1976; Supplement 1977, compiled by Nancy K. Taylor.

Sorenson, James R. "Biomedical Innovation, Uncertainty, and Doctor-Patient Interaction," *Jounal of Health and Social Behavior* 15 (December, 1974): 366-74.

Steinfels, Peter, and Robert M. Veatch, eds. *Death Inside Out.* New York: Haper & Row, 1975.

Sullivan, Michael T. "The Dying Person — IIis Plight and His Right." *New England Law Review* 8 (1973): 197-216.

Thomson, Judith Jarvis. "Rights and Deaths." *Philosophy & Public Affairs* 2 (1973): 146-159.

_____. "Killing, Letting Die, and the Trolley Problem," *The Monist* 59 (1976): 204-17.

Tolstoy, Leo. *Death of Ivan Ilych.* New York: Signet Books, New American Library, 1960.

Toynbee, Arnold, et al. *Man's Concern with Death.* New York: McGraw-Hill, 1968.

Twycross, R. G. "The Use of Narcotic Analgesics in Terminal Illness," *Journal of Medical Ethics* 1 (April, 1975): 1071.

_____. "Clinical Experience with Diamorphine in Advanced Malignant Disease," *International J. of Clinical Pharmocology, Therapy, and Toxicology* 9 (1974): 184-98.

Veatch, Robert M. "Brain Death: Welcome Definition of Dangerous

Judgment?" *Hastings Center Report* 2 (November 1972): 40-43.
_____. "Choosing Not to Prolong Dying," *Medical Dimensions*,
December, 1972, pp. 8-10 ff.
_____. *Death, Dying, and the Biological Revolution*. New Haven:
Yale University Press, 1976.
Vodiga, B. "Euthanasia and The Right to Die." *Chicago-Kent Law Review* 51 (1974): 1-40.
Wassmer, Thomas A. "Between Life and Death: Ethical and Moral
Issues Involved in Recent Medical Advances." *Villanova Law
Review* 13 (1968): 759-83.
White, Laurens P., ed. "Care of Patients with Fatal Illness." *Annals of
the New York Academy of Sciences* 164 (December, 1969):
635-896.
White, Robert B., and H. Tristram Engelhardt, Jr. "Case Studies in
Bioethics: A Demand to Die," *Hastings Center Report* 5 (June
1975): 9 ff.
Williams, Robert H., ed. *To Live and To Die: When, Why, and How*. New
York: Springer-Verlag, 1973.
Worcester, Alfred. *The Care of the Aging, the Dying, and the Dead*. 2nd
ed. Springfield, Ill.: Charles C. Thomas, 1961.

NOTES ON CONTRIBUTORS

Michael D. Bayles, Ph.D., Professor of Philosophy, University of Kentucky.

H. Tristram Engelhardt, Jr., M.D., Ph.D., Rosemary Kennedy Professor of the Philosophy of Medicine, Kennedy Institute, Center for Bioethics, Georgetown University.

Samuel Gorovitz, Ph.D., Professor and Chairman, Department of Philosophy, University of Maryland.

Dallas M. High, Ph.D., Professor of Philosophy, University of Kentucky.

Robert P. Hudson, M.D., Chairman, Department of the History and Philosophy of Medicine, The University of Kansas Medical Center.

John Ladd, Ph.D., Professor of Philosophy, Brown University.

James F. Toole, M.D., L.L.B., The Walter C. Teagle Professor of Neurology, The Bowman Gray School of Medicine of Wake Forest University.

Robert M. Veatch, Ph.D., Senior Associate, Hastings Center of the Institute of Society, Ethics and the Life Sciences.